NURSES

Pulling Together To Make A Difference

Venner M. Farley Ed.D., R.N.

toExcel
San Jose New York Lincoln Shanghai

Pulling Together to Make a Difference

Published by toExcel
an imprint of iUniverse.com, Inc.

For information address:
iUniverse.com, Inc.
620 North 48th Street
Suite 201
Lincoln, NE 68504-3467
www.iuniverse.com

ISBN: 0-595-00539-X

Printed in the United States of America

Dedication

For Dee... Steadfast and True

Acknowledgments

Thanks to Laura Gasparis Vonfrolio, RN, PhD, CEN, CCRN for
her generous and empowering spirit. Thanks to the staff at Power
Publications for their support and thanks to Cheryl DeCicco who
turned my tapes into manuscripts,and finally into this book.

NURSES PULLING TOGETHER TO MAKE A DIFFERENCE

Preface

All nurses need exceptional leadership skills today in order to transport our profession forward, despite the resource constraints plaguing all health care organizations. All nurses must participate in the creation of standards of care that achieve quality, are cost effective, and can be rationally implemented. We must work together to create work environments that foster professional practice, maintain quality outcomes, and are cost effective. To achieve these goals, nurses must become masters of change and transformational leaders, willing to be empowered themselves, and willing to empower other nurses.

Nurses must recognize the inherent responsibilities of leadership in all professional nursing practice today. It will take great commitment on the part of all registered nurses to realize that a revolutionary health care environment will be with us for awhile, and that we must all cope with the economics of health care as they exist today in terms of "do more with less, but do it nicer."

Since all nurses manage patient care and since all nurses must readily accept the legal, ethical, and moral responsibility inherent in our practice, it is not a gigantic leap for nurses to recognize their innate leadership responsibility for resource consciousness. We must move on, then, to accept our responsibilities regarding bottom line management. Nurses must take the lead in interpreting this concept for all healthcare workers: our colleague physicians, our colleague nurses, and all ancillary personnel. In the future we will all need to give more, and do better, with fewer resources. It has often been said that we all need to work smarter, not harder.

At the same time that we are concerned as nurse leaders with optimizing quality outcomes and cost effectiveness, we must be equally concerned with reframing and reshaping nursing's work. Constant change is the order of the day in health care delivery, and this is especially true in the nursing profession. Therefore, preparing nurse leaders to be change masters is critical. We have only seen the tip of the iceberg as regards the amount of change that must take place in the health care delivery system in order for there to be a universal access system that works for United States citizens. Nurse leaders understand that the refreezing aspect of the change process has evaporated, and that the only part of change that we can count on is its rapidity and its constancy. Predictable uncertainty is the order of the day in health care delivery and it is also the element in change mastering that reveals ones commitment to being a change agent. Managing change therefore, is a critical component of every nurse leader's repertoire.

NURSES MAKING A DIFFERENCE

QUALITY

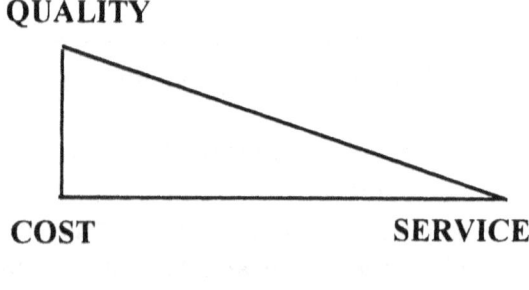

COST   **SERVICE**

OUR 3 CHALLENGES

Chapter One

MANAGE THINGS...LEAD PEOPLE

Management has been defined as "doing things right." Whereas leadership has been defined as " doing the right things." Since most nurses become managers because they were good nurses, many nurses in management positions lack training in the science of management/leadership. There are twelve qualities that all leaders must have:

1) A leader has a mission that matters, and performs as if that mission matters;
2) A leader is very ethical;
3) A leader is a big thinker;
4) A leader is a change-master;
5) A leader is sensitive to other people;
6) A leader is a risk-taker;
7) A leader is a decision-maker;
8) A leader uses power and political skill;
9) A leader communicates effectively;
10) A leader believes in and is a team-builder;
11) A leader is courageous;
12) A leader is committed (Bethel, 1990).

The study and practice of these qualities of leadership are integral to the role. It is only after the managerial skills are mastered that those managerial skills can develop into leadership skills. For example, the new manager must develop the skills of: directing, creative thinking, decision-making, listening, constructive criticism, problem-solving, and implementing technology. With experience, the nurse manager will move into another level in terms of skill evolution. (Renesch, 1992). Leadership is a higher level of skill evolution than is management. Leadership skills that evolve from managerial skills are: supporting instead of directing; inspiring creativity instead of creatively thinking; delegating instead of making decisions; ensuring understanding instead of simply listening; resolving conflict instead of offering constructive criticism; and humanizing technology instead of simply implementing technology.

Table 1
ROLES OF MANAGER VS LEADER

OLD MANAGER	LEADER
• ADMINISTERS	• INNOVATES
• ...IS A COPY	• ...IS AN ORIGINAL
• FOCUSES ON SYSTEM & STRUCTURE	• FOCUSES ON PEOPLE
• RELIES ON CONTROL	• INSPIRES TRUST
• SHORT RANGE PERSPECTIVE	• LONG RANGE PLANNING
• ASKS HOW & WHEN	• ASKS WHY
• EYE ON BOTTOM LINE	• EYE ON HORIZON
• IMITATES	• ORIGINATES
• ACCEPTS STATUS QUO	• CHALLENGES STATUS QUO
• CLASSIC "GOOD SOLDIER"	• HIS/HER OWN PERSON
• DOES THINGS RIGHT	• DOES THE RIGHT THING

It should be clear in the nurse manager's/leader's mind that the most important element s/he brings to leadership in nursing is service to the nurses who get the work done.

President Eisenhower once defined leadership as "the ability to get someone to do what you want them to do, when you want them to do it without them knowing that that's what you wanted them to do." In the 21st century there are parts of this definition which will be history. However, the charismatic leader will always be able to do just that. In truth, there are very few charismatic leaders in nursing. The great need in nursing is to develop inspirational leaders who are truly charismatic; and who have a clear vision of the future and the ability to move the profession forward.

Table 2

TANGIBLE SKILLS OF NURSING MANAGERS	INTANGIBLE SKILLS OF NURSING MANAGERS
• PLANNING	• BELIEFS
• ORGANIZING	• VALUES
• CONTROLLING	• IDEALS
• EVALUATING	• DECISION-MAKING
• SYSTEMS VIEWPOINT	• JUDGMENT
• HUMAN MANAGEMENT	• INTEGRATING SKILLS
• FLEXIBILITY/NEGOTIATION/ COMPROMISE	• POLITICAL SKILL
• NURSING KNOWLEDGE	• ANALYTIC THINKING
• HEALTH KNOWLEDGE	• VISION

To make the difference that the title of this book purports to have as its goal means to recognize the main ingredients of service to the nurses who get the work done. First and foremost there must be a willingness in the leader to serve other people. Second, there must be an understanding of the kind and quality of service that needs to be given. Inherent in both of these stipulations is the understanding that service is an attitude, and that attitudes are the things we most deeply believe. Criticism frequently leveled at nurse managers is that they do not care about the working nurse. That once elevated into the position of nurse manager, the organization becomes the be all and end all. At the present time there is no bigger buzz word than "quality service" in all service industries today. Nurse leaders have to internalize that concept so that they first exhibit quality service to the nurses who work with them, and that the symbol of quality service is carried forth from the very top in the organization.

A new nurse leader may legitimately ask "how do I serve my people", and the answer comes back, "serve them with sensitivity," i.e., treat them as you would like to be treated so that they will turn around and serve others in exactly the same way. Those "others" are other nurses, colleague physicians, and, certainly and most importantly, patients and their families. True leaders never forget that there is a direct correlation between the way they serve the people with whom they work and the way the followers serve others.

Historically, managers manage things; and leaders lead people. Both of these capabilities are essential for nurses in managerial/leadership roles today. Managers work with and through people to meet organizational goals. Leaders attempt to influence human behavior, irrespective of the goal. Leadership, then, is influencing people so that they wish to meet the organizational goals. Nurse leaders inspire the nurse at the practice level to recognize the innate professionalism of the work that nurses do. They help the working nurse to understand that it is not the job s/he does... but how s/he does the job... that entitles the registered nurse to be called a professional.

Few nurses go to work intending to perform poorly. But the pressures extant on the registered nurse today are enormous, and the rewards are fewer than they've ever been -even though salaries have improved. Therefore, leaders must, by their example, show registered nurses how to pursue excellence...in a time of predictable uncertainty and cost containment. (see tables 1 & 2).

It is incumbent upon the nurse leader to assist the working nurse to adjust to the pressures in health care delivery today: rising competition, and what this means to every health care agency; prospective payment systems;

managed care in its multiple definitions; increasingly sophisticated medical technology with a very high price tag; changing providers, including the changing practice of the physician; the changing patient; substitute products and services for client care; and the changing practice of nursing itself. (see tables 3,4,5)

Table 3 **THE CURRENT HEALTH CARE ENVIRONMENT**

<u>OLD</u>	<u>NEW</u>
• Focus on current operations in the organization	• Highly Competitive
• Addresses internal contentions and conflict	• Very Technological
• Very narrow view of organizational structure and development	• Managed Care
• Very tight controls and highly bureaucratic	• Focus on Internal & External Customers

NURSING VALUES IN A RESTRUCTURED
Table 4 **HEALTH CARE SYSTEM**

<u>HEALTH CARE SYSTEM</u>	<u>NURSING VALUES</u>
• Competition	• Recognition and rewards
• Managed Care	• Leadership support
• High Cost technology	• Career Opportunities
• Organizational complexity	• Shared governance and professional practice
• Cost consciousness	• Collaboration in clinical practice
• Physicians control	• Advanced practice and provision of primary care

Table 5 **EVOLVING SKILLS**

<u>NURSING MANAGEMENT</u>	<u>NURSING LEADERSHIP</u>
• Directing	• Supporting
• Creative thinking	• Inspiring Creativity
• Decision making	• Delegating
• Listening	• Ensuring understanding
• Constructive criticism	• Enhancing others
• Problem solving	• Resolving conflict
• Implementing technology	• Humanizing technology
THINGS	PEOPLE

4

Chapter Two

THE ETCHED-IN-STONE SYNDROME:
BECOMING A CHANGE AGENT.

The cost of health care in this country exceeds $ 900 billion a year. Since the onset of prospective payment in 1982 the "pie" of health care has been getting smaller. So in order for health care agencies and organizations to make a profit anywhere near the profit they made prior to 1982, their piece of the pie must get bigger. This means, unquestionably, that competition is the name of the game in health care today. Competition has not decreased the cost of health care. There is no question that the American health care system is on the verge of the greatest changes since the onset of Medicare in 1964. Presently, health care costs in excess of 16% of the gross domestic product (GDP). This makes health care the second largest industry in the United States.

All health care systems, which we used to call hospitals, are concerned about their payor mix. It is critical that health care agencies have a satisfactory payor mix in order to keep their slice of the pie commensurate with what they need to pay the bills.

For example, in normal, every day averages Medicaid pays a health care organization about 80 cents for every dollar of health care spent on a medicaid patient. Medicare pays about 97 cents for every dollar for health care cost to a Medicare patient. Contracts, often called managed care, in health care today, pay the health care agency about $ 1.12 for every dollar of health care cost spent. And finally the indemnity plans, which are only about 20% of insurance policies today, pay the health care agency about $ 1.60 to $ 1.90 per dollar of health care cost spent on the patient. Evidently, hospitals must have a sufficient number of patients who contracted i.e., managed care patients, or indemnity plan payors so that they are in the black, at least some of the time. A cursory analysis would indicate that if the bulk of an agency's patients are medicaid and medicare, that agency will constantly run in the red. Competition means that the health care organizations we used to call hospitals are in a constant battle of merchandising themselves; and increasing their merchandise portfolio.

The pressures in health care today are;
1. Rising competition on all fronts;
2. The everlastingness of prospective payment systems;
3. Managed care as an entity for discounting health care;
4. Increased technology so sophisticated it requires a very high price tag

5. The changing health care provider, for example, the physician and changing patterns of practice;
6. The change in the patient who is very savvy, and intelligent about health care costs and is not opposed to "shopping";
7. Substitute products and services;
8. The changing nurse. (<u>Modern Health Care</u>, '92-94)

Obviously, we are in a time of revolutionary change in health care in the United States. Needless to say, everyone resists change. And in the 1990s as regards health care, it is true to say that the only thing we can count on is predictable uncertainty. Therefore, adjusting and accommodating to change is an essential ingredient in leadership at all levels of nursing practice at this time. Dr. Kubler-Ross (1969), years ago, described the stages of death and dying as being:

1. **Denial**
2. **Anger**
3. **Bargaining**
4. **Depression**
5. **Acceptance**

This model can also be used in describing resistance to change. For example: since it is common knowledge that everyone resists change, it is natural to expect that everyone involved in change immediately goes into denial. Denial means that we refuse to accept and/or acknowledge the change itself. As Kubler-Ross said, many people never leave denial. This is true also in change processing. Those who do get out of denial, go into anger, which means they are very irritated with the possibility of change. It could even be described as "mad as hell and not going to take it anymore." Those few who come out of anger, go into bargaining which is a very short stage and not very productive: "if you do this then I'll do that." Those people who go into bargaining come out of it fast, and go into depression. The state of depression, as regards change, is a very serious state of melancholia characterized by decreased energy. The people who are depressed regarding change are actually immobilized. Very few people who go into depression in change processing come out of it. But those few who do come out of depression go into acceptance. It would however, be erroneous to consider acceptance a happy state. Rather it is simply the acknowledgement of the fact that the change is going to occur and "we might as well adjust." So even acceptance is not a happy state. However, it needs to be acknowledged that acceptance is the state in which the leader can begin to work with participants, either to reach a negotiated accommodation, or to enter an actual planning phase to begin to process the change effectively. (Kubler-Ross 1969).

Acceptance then, becomes resignation and can be considered the "readiness" state for processing change.

Table 6

STAGES OF CHANGE NURSE LEADER BEHAVIORS

Denial. Empathic and nonjudgmental. Use good listening skills.
Anger. Acknowledge feelings, continue to listen, but be assertive, utilizing problem solving skills.
Bargaining. Attempt to bring real problems into the open and utilize negotiation skills to get all you need when you can't get all you want.
Depression. Provide information, acknowledge the pain, utilize patience see into the long-term.
Acceptance. Acknowledge resignation, provide more information, be directive as needed, assign tasks and monitor those tasks, and accept readiness as a time to provide further direction and guidelines.
Adapted From: Perlman, *Nursing Management* - April 1990

Rosabeth Moss-Kanter (1989), from Harvard has said that it takes three years for a major change process to come to fruition. It is unfortunate that nurse leaders, in my experience, have never had that much time to accommodate any change. However, revolution - of itself - means change; and assisting others to adapt to change is critical, if nursing is to take its place in the reform of health care that will occur in this century.

Managing change for nurse leaders is often the most frustrating, exasperating, and often unsuccessful activity of leadership. In fact, 75% of the people who initiate changes stop them because of resistance and never get beyond resistance itself (Kanter).

It may be helpful to use someone else's philosophy in developing our own philosophy regarding change in a revolutionary environment:

We shift priorities, then rules, make rules up - whatever it takes. Our mission, our challenge, is to stop reacting to the backlash and start riding the waves of change. The sharp edges of the hierarchy must yield to the softer curves of cooperation and collegiality. Skepticism is rampant. What has been, is now dysfunctional; what will be, has not yet taken shape. Letting go of things that have worked before, is not easy. Stepping forward with confidence demands a transitional leader who dares to be different. The transitional leader accepts this challenge as an opportunity to go beyond the realities of the past to the possibilities of the future. What has been, will never be again. What is, no longer works. What will be, is now taking shape. Each of us shares the opportunity to become an architect of the future: a transitional leader (Source: Leadership In Transition by Neis and Kingdon, 1990).

There are three sources of change:
1) Trauma

2) Design (productive change designed by leaders); and

3) The passage of time.

Leaders in nursing need to ask themselves these questions:

1. At what level do I resist change?

2. At what issues do I resist change?

Leaders must do for themselves what they would like the staff nurse to do also: Let go of whole ideas; let go of old concepts and resentments; and let go of unuseful attitudes. William James, one of the greatest psychologists of the early 20th century, has said "when you change your attitude, you change your life." This is the very essence of leadership in change, for when a leader changes his or her attitude, s/he not only changes h/his life but also changes the lives of everyone who works with that leader.

Figure 1

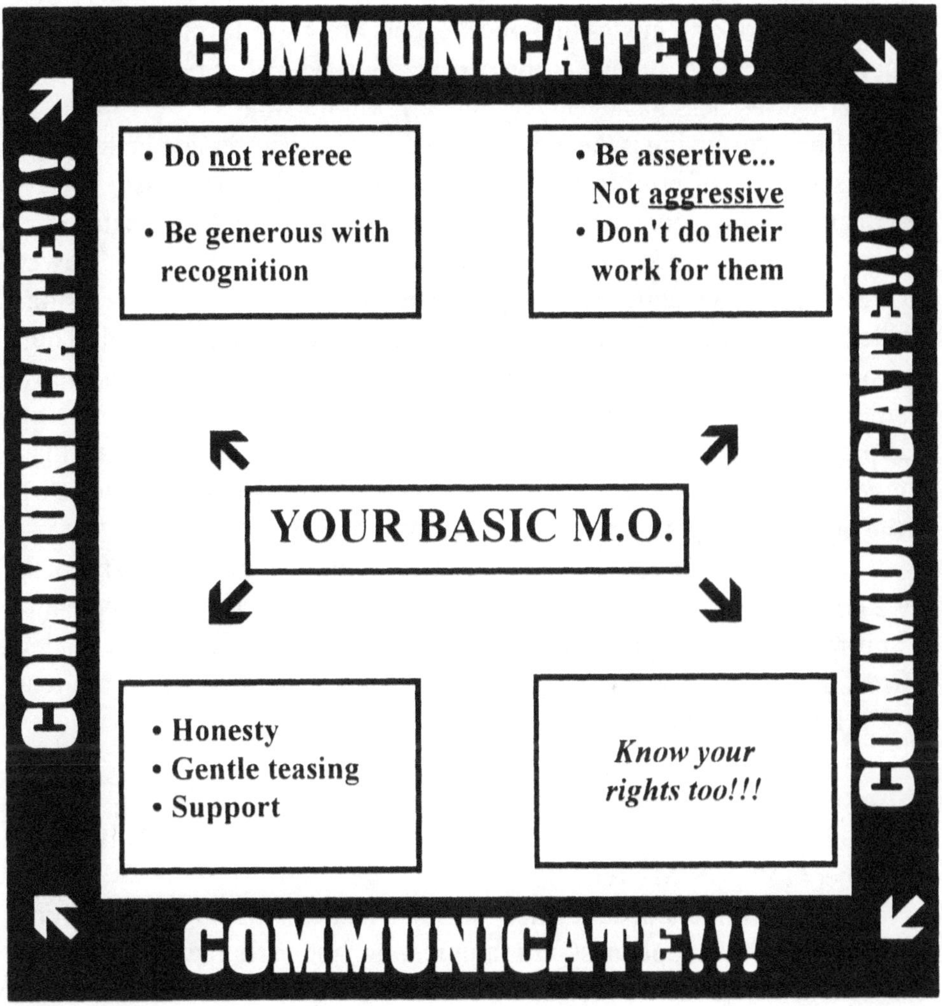

COMMUNICATE!!!

- Do **not** referee

- Be generous with recognition

- Be assertive...
  Not **aggressive**
- Don't do their work for them

YOUR BASIC M.O.

- Honesty
- Gentle teasing
- Support

Know your rights too!!!

COMMUNICATE!!!

This naturally leads to the concept of empowerment. Empowerment has become a buzz word in nursing, which very few nurses really understand. Empowerment means giving power to others who operate at a disadvantage in the organization (Vogt & Murrell, 1990). It is common knowledge among working nurses that once leaders are given formal power, they forget the people who work in the organization who are greatly disadvantaged. Powerlessness has been very powerful in nursing.

Because nursing is the most female dominated profession in this country, nurses have suffered from the same problems of antifeminism and paternalism as has society itself. Women in the United States historically, even hysterically, have suffered from inferiority complexes because of powerlessness. The consequences of powerlessness are low morale, small mindedness, bureaucratic domination, and tight territorial control. These are common behavioral characteristics of nurse leaders in formal powerful positions in nursing i.e., directors of nursing, assistant directors of nursing, vice presidents of nursing. These formal leaders in nursing have been loath to give up their own power by building, developing and increasing the power of the practicing registered nurse. This must change.

We can no longer use empowerment or empowering as buzz words, if we do not intend to assess their relationship to the forward movement of the profession of nursing. There are four key assessments for all leaders (formal and informal) in nursing to utilize within their own environment:
1. Am I making a difference, what impact am I having?
2. Do I have the requisite skills, do I have the ability?
3. Am I making a significant contribution in terms of meaning?
4. Am I heading in the right direction, that is, am I growing in a satisfactory manner? (Vogt & Merrell, 1990).

Empowerment occurs when the nurse leader is willing to share h/his power through trust, openness, communication, and participation in the formal systems of the institution. Some of these will grow into commitment to the institution. A sense of personal worth contributes to personal self-fulfillment. In other words, empowerment results in personal as well as organizational well being. Leaders need to react positively, rather than defensively to these new realities. An empowerment orientation says "if we can have happy workers, if we can facilitate the individual to be productive and participative in the working environment, the organization is advantaged." Enabling registered nurses to become self-initiated professionals who are recognized as an important part of the institution is the single most important activity of nurse leaders today. This is the dominant change that must be accomplished, and go far beyond simple lip service.

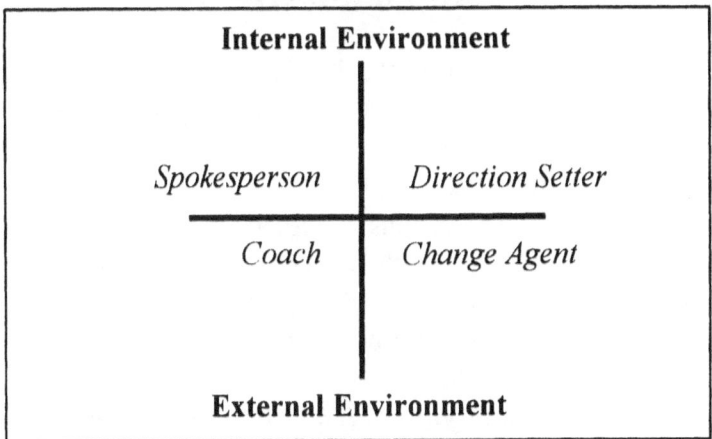

Figure 2

LEADER'S ROLES

	Internal Environment	
Spokesperson		*Direction Setter*
Coach		*Change Agent*
	External Environment	

We must move away from the "etched in stone syndrome" and sacrifice sacred cows in nursing, for it is true that registered nurses have been overmanaged and underled. We must not fall victim to the traps of resisting change that have been part of the profession from its beginning. Some of those traps which must be eliminated are:

1. Using yesterday's solution for today's problem
2. Assuming present trends are temporary
3. Neglecting opportunities of future change
4. Resisting a sense of humor
5. Expecting to succeed without requisite effort
6. The absence of a personal coping strategy (Bethel, 1990).

Chapter Three
LEADERSHIP MANDATES NOW

Nursing leaders must foster the development of visions, values, and strategies in the nursing profession. A leader is a big thinker who forces, inspires, attracts, creates and changes. A leader is one who serves us by making a difference, being energetic, by encouragement, by creativity, enthusiasm and imagination. The visions, values and strategies that each nursing organization must build on are: the concept of service; cooperation; encouragement; quality; rewards; recognition; integrity; leadership; applied clinical research; and full partnerships on the part of all members in the nursing organization to build the future.

Alvin Toffler stated in _Power Shift_ (1990) that power must shift to the participation of all members of the organization, each having equal amounts of power... that is the ability to create change. Without this energy that equalizes power among all members, crisis management continues. Crisis management consists of putting out fires without planning for the future; and it is reactive. It does not depend on foresight but rather depends on no sight, that is no vision at all. Crisis management results in confusion for all workers within the institution. Crisis results in conflict which is very difficult to manage. The stress of crisis is not often thought about by nurse leaders; but it is so crucial, that it must be talked about in the dynamic and complex world of health care delivery today. Nurses working in health care centers today see the crisis of alienation (Vogt & Murrell, 1990). The crisis of alienation means that nurses feel an un-belonging-ness to the organization: organizational aversion on the part of the practicing nurse. This aversion is manifested by conflict, rumor and innuendo. It can be managed by improving the right of the staff nurses to self-esteem and positive self-regard, thereby decreasing alienation, decreasing stress, and promoting a sense of empowerment which conquers alienation.

In truth, the leader's role in empowerment is even greater than it is in more traditional roles. Sharing responsibility and empowering others does not mean giving up the leadership role. On the contrary, it actually means a higher level of morality, a higher level of ethical practice, and a higher level of human competence in all the roles of leadership (Vogt & Murrell, 1990).

Practicing nurses are information starved. They have never known the truth of what goes on in the bureaucratic organization; and they have not trusted the hierarchy. The leader's role in empowerment means shifting those attitudes which have deprived nurses of the ability to create change within themselves and within their organizations. It is also the leader's role to redefine the leadership role in the empowered organization, and to use crises as opportunities to take risks in planning for the future. The leader in an empowered organization has the same responsibilities of informing, deciding, planning, evaluating, motivating, and developing as in more traditional structures. However, the focus of the leader in empowering other members of the staff is to develop synergy on the part of all members within the organization. Synergy is the state in which the whole is more than the sum of the parts. Using the synergistic approach (recommended by Stephen Covey, 1991) means that the leader and the staff nurses are change catalysts together. They can assess every situation; they can analyze together; and they can be amazingly productive and creative; using both their right and left brain as the situation demands.

They are not in competition with each other. They are not in conflict with each other, and therefore they can focus on the best possible means of utilizing their combined intelligence to meet the visions, the values and the strategies of the organization in these revolutionary times (Pinchot, 1993).

How do you rate as an empowered leader?
1. Do you encourage participation by others?
2. Do you give power away by enabling others to create change?
3. In your organization does the nursing division have a written mission statement, a written statement of visions, a written statement of values? ... a written strategic plan?
4. Do you question yourself?
5. Do you have an awareness of how to improve or increase loyalties within the division of nursing?
6. Do you compete fairly with other nurses?
7. Do you have a high tolerance for frustration?
8. Do you lose without pouting?
9. Do you control the impulse to get even?
10. Do you stay alert for new ideas even when they come from other people?
11. Do you acknowledge good ideas when they come from other people?
12. Is there a reward system in your institution for staff nurses? Is there a recognition program in your institution for staff nurses?
    (Bethel; Vogt & Murrell)

"Perhaps the most important lesson for the professional manager is that the professional manager is a servant. Rank does not confer privilege or give power. It imposes responsibility". *Peter Drucker*

Chapter Four

CURING PSYCHOSCLEROSIS

Lao-Tse, an ancient Chinese philosopher wrote, "a leader is one who serves." Service is an attitude. Behavior is what we say and do; but attitudes are what we think and feel. A leader is one who serves because s/he have the willingness and ability to serve others and understand the type, kind and quality of service to be given.

It will be no surprise to most nurses that nurses are promoted to managerial positions, not because they are good managers, but because they are good nurses. The two are not necessarily the same. Until recent years, most nurse managers were not prepared for managerial positions. Many nurses have the innate ability to be leaders; but all nurse managers and leaders need additional preparation.

Psychosclerosis is "hardening of the attitudes." This condition is endemic in the nursing profession. An effective nurse leader cannot have this condition. It must be cured in every manager/leader for the manager/leader to succeed. The cure for *Psychosclerosis* in nurse leaders is to develop sensitivity. Sensitivity is the willingness to treat other nurses the way you would like to be treated, not the way you have been treated. Nurses, by and large, have grown up in a heritage punishment based on the diploma school model of obedience first and above all else, and discipline secondary to obedience. But being held prisoners by our heredity and environment leads to *Psychosclerosis*...not to successful leadership.

It is the leader's purpose to move people from one type of readiness to another type of readiness, depending on the situation and type of change involved. This is why it is so important for leaders to have sensitivity: to interpret where a person is and to move them along the continuum of readiness for change. The importance of sensitivity cannot be overemphasized in your effectiveness as a leader.

Nurses are ready for the inspiration of leadership. It is true that, like people in all occupations and professions: some are able and willing; some are able and not willing; some are willing and not able; some are neither willing nor able.

But leadership - charismatic and inspirational- can bring nurses into the 21st century with a sense of self worth that has been sorely lacking. Hardening of the attitudes - *Psychosclerosis* -has been the result of that ab-

sence. Treating, and then eliminating, this condition begins with role identification and pride in one's work. Strategies of salvation in this treatment
involves having enough information to be organizationally aware of one's
own duties and the duties of others in the system.

The following role delineations will help in clarifying professional
accountabilities:

Table 7

WHAT I OWE THE BOSS	WHAT THE BOSS OWES ME
1. Performance	1. Direction
2. Information	2. Information
3. Requests	3. Support
4. Patience	4. Feedback
5. Commitment to the Boss's goals	5. Strategic planning
6. Courage and self discipline	6. Inspiration & encouragement
7. Respect	7. Discipline and correction

WHAT NO ONE OWES ANYONE
1. Mind reading
2. Psychoanalysis
3. Personal affection
4. Allegiance to the same values
5. Self-sacrifice
6. Perfection

In other words, we are each in charge of ourselves. Although everyone resists change, it is possible to decrease resistance to change by understanding natural responses to change in terms of stress, fear and doubt. Understanding the concepts of what I owe the boss, what the boss owes me, and
what no one owes anyone, will decrease the amount of distress that is in-
curred during any change process.

Psychosclerosis is hardening of the attitudes. The earliest history for
nurses in the United States is entwined with a heritage of punishment, a
culture of poverty, and a culture of negativity. It is almost as if nurses took
vows of obedience, poverty, and powerlessness. We have never recognized
the power of that powerlessness. We have never realized that nursing has
come a long way from the Nightingale training schools that honored obedience and discipline and powerlessness above all else.

The question to ask of one's self is, if attitudes were contagious . . .
would you want someone to catch yours? If the answer is "no," there is work

to be done. Winston Churchill once said that, "an optimist sees an opportunity in every calamity, a pessimist sees the calamity in every opportunity." The latter statement (pessimist) is a very good definition of someone with *Psychosclerosis.*

Here is a list of *Psychosclerotic* behaviors:
• Competing instead of collaborating
• Operating autonomously rather than cooperatively
• Blaming . . . and justifying
• Bickering . . . and quarreling
• Lack of trust
• Excusitis
• Inconsistency
• Conflicting goals

Managers/leaders in nursing must be willing to place their major emphasis on interpersonal relationships at work. For team building, and in order to manage interpersonal relationships in human resources, the leader must be willing to manage self; manage work; manage people; manage relations; and manage situations. Of course this means handling situations and behaviors through problem solving and decision-making; through increasing motivation, cooperation and team work; while stressing that role modeling, personal example, and personal accountability (with a positive mental attitude) is job one.

If the nurse leader makes curing *Psychosclerosis* a primary objective, the self-managed nursing team can become a reality, and the teams will be:

T	**Terrifically**
E	**Energized**
A	**And**
M	**Motivated**

Chapter Five

NURSING IS ON THE BRINK OF GREAT REFORM

I believe in myself and in my nursing colleagues. And more importantly, I believe that nursing is on the brink of its greatest growth ever. When compared to Erickson's developmental stages nursing as a profession is just like any other adolescent... still seeking its own unique identity. Based on our dysfunctional history of an "heritage of punishment" where obedience and discipline were valued above all else in the Nightingale-like schools of nursing, we have failed to thrive and move into adulthood. We have failed to move to the stages of autonomy and true accountability. Therefore, nursing has arrived at the end of the 20th century as an anonymous profession with a diminished capacity compared to our physician colleagues; and an adolescent propensity to set the blame instead of solving the problem.

Individually and collectively, we are ready to thrive. Actually we are being forced to move by the incredible changes occurring all around us in the health care reform revolution. If we do not change, our profession will not survive. Therefore, I believe in nursing as a professional discipline, different from but complementary to, "physicianing." I believe we, as nurses, must be autonomous in our practice and equally as important, that we must be accountable to our clients for that essential health care service called nursing, which clients and families need and only nurses can provide. Change is the order of the day in nursing, in society, and throughout the health care industry. Stability is an illusion. In one way or another, we are all affected by societal, organizational, structural, and political changes. These changes involve technology, standards of practice, reimbursement, etc.

Resisting change may be natural, but it is also a natural human failing. There is nothing more important to the profession of nursing today than our excitement about the prospects of change for nursing, and nurses; and our commitment as individual nurses to the implementation of those changes.

These times of predictable uncertainty for the health care industry, and for health care consumers must be viewed as opportunities for our professional membership. Never has there been more opportunity for prosperity for nurses and for the profession of nursing. It is true that the revolution we are in will exist for many years. However nursing must be in the forefront, as the gatekeeper for health care delivery, as the new system of health care delivery evolves.

Now is our time, as professionals, to move from self indulgence to self discipline. It is time to share with each other the truth of nursing's mission. It is time to work in partnership with our physician colleagues, the health care consumer, and all aspects of the new health care delivery system's administration.

Finances in health care organizations will continue to be constricted for the remainder of our careers. There will be new forms of competition arriving at incredible rates of speed. The rapid changes we have begun to see will continue for as long as we live. Health care reform is a process and a journey which will take many years, predictably well into the 21st century. The style of today's nursing leader must match that rapid change. Today's nursing leader must be active and intrusive, recognizing that true leadership is transformational today; and epitomized by the ability to look at the same things as everybody else and see something different. Nursing leaders today must be characterized by their willingness and ability to color outside the lines.

It is time to move away from nursing's ancient history as the handmaiden to the physician; and of nursing as a dependent occupation. For all of my years as a registered nurse I have longed for nursing to finally reach maturity...and what we witness today is a significant step into that new, mature future. I will ask an interesting question: Would Florence Nightingale agree with me? Let me recall for you her motto: "Create and do not criticize." Florence wrote that "Every great reformer began by being a solitary dissenter-but in every case it was a positive dissent; ending not in protest but in great reform" (Ulrich, 1992).

Nursing is indeed ready for great reform. Our history has been characterized by three S's: self-sacrifice, submissiveness, and self-effacement. Let us affirm that the past is past. We must create a professional impact that clearly defines nursing as transformed and ready for these new challenges. Just like Florence Nightingale, we must be tough, canny, powerful, autonomous, and even heroic.

Figure 3

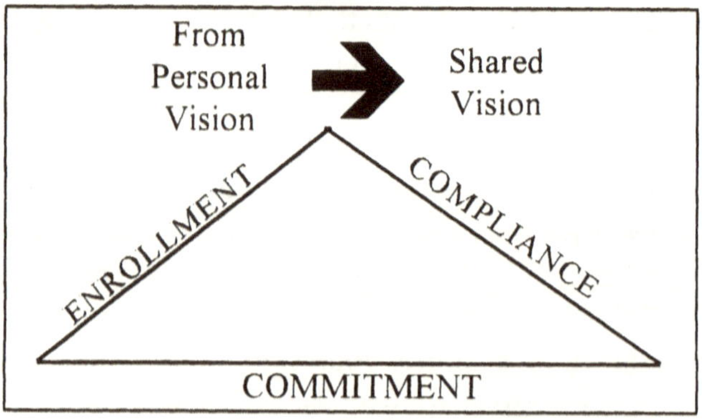

From Personal Vision → Shared Vision

ENROLLMENT

COMPLIANCE

COMMITMENT

Chapter Six

SURVIVAL STRATEGIES

We are all affected by the organizational and structural changes occurring in, around and within the health care industry. Health care trends for this last decade of the 20th century, and surely for the first decades of the 21st century are:

- soaring health care expenditures
- hospital closures
- population shifts
- changes in physician and nursing practice
- shift to ambulatory care
- growth in managed care
- technological advances
- emphasis on quality
- emphasis on service
- emphasis on cost containment
- challenges regarding work force needs
- challenges regarding work force shortages (Lathrop, 1993).

This is not an exclusive list. It simply enumerates the most current changes occurring in health care, and the trends that will most affect the future of health care delivery for the foreseeable future.

To resist change is a human failing. Resistance to change is to be expected and must be managed for change to actually occur. To be successful in nursing, we must recognize the need for change, we must develop the ability to implement change, and we must ourselves adapt to these changes. There will be nothing more important in securing the successful implementation of change in our health care systems than our excitement about the prospects of change; and our commitment as individuals to the implementation of those changes. A list of examples for the future of nursing in health care delivery regarding such changes, include these:

- achievement of outcomes
- financial integrity
- willingness to adapt to change
- increased productivity
- cost control in delivery
- service to our customers
- quality in our service

It is easy to conclude that the tenents for the future of nursing are congruent with health care trends in general.

Robert Bramson (1981), a Berkeley-based organizational psychologist, has compared Dr. Kubler-Ross' grieving process to what happens as human factors impede change implementation. Dr. Bramson has placed resistance to change in the same categories that Dr. Ross placed her grieving factors: *Stage one: Denial and Isolation:* initial feelings of "this can't be true" and a focus on self deception. *Stage two: Anger:* when the first stage of denial cannot be maintained longer, feelings give way to anger, envy, and resentment. *Stage three: Bargaining:* this phase is always short-lived. It may postpone the inevitable...but briefly. This phase delays acceptance and realistic action. *Stage four: Depression:* when the need for change can no longer effectively be denied, and bargaining has not worked, then anger is replaced with a sense of enormous loss. The result of these feelings of helplessness and loss is depression. During the depression phase, calls to action are premature. *Stage five: Resignation:* This phase has sometimes been called acceptance. However acceptance implies some kind of enthusiasm. Actually resignation is the appropriate word because it comes with time, as individuals and organizations work through the stages of grieving. Resignation simply means that the process can now be facilitated with support and understanding; but it cannot be accessed rapidly. Resignation may be followed by acceptance, but neither resignation nor acceptance should be mistaken for happy stages. They simply provide the base on which individuals can begin to act in implementing change.

Nurses sometimes do not put into practice what they know intellectually. Becoming a change agent takes planning...it is not accidental. We may teach change theory very well, but not use that change theory in real life as we implement change. The first and most serious difficulty in implementing change is dealing with resistance; and the fact that we do not plan for handling resistance. This is the most neglected aspect of developing a change process. If there is always resistance to change, then intellectually we need to know where resistance starts. Resistance frequently begins with the behavior of the change agent who does not focus on communication, involvement, participation.

When the people who are to be affected by the change begin to buy-in to the change because they understand its effects on their personal life, then their need to maintain the status quo may diminish. Commitment to change must always be preceded by information-giving, and buy-in must always be preceded by involvement. So buy-in and involvement result in

20

commitment.

Therefore, expect resistance; and most importantly...plan for it (Kanter, 1989). Success in implementing change requires several ingredients. If we are to succeed in describing a change plan and then implementing it, there has to be a strong need for change. Certainly there has never been a stronger need for change in health care delivery than there is now.

There has to be readiness for change. And the great work of leadership in transformation and transition will be preparing nurses in the work setting for these changes. Admittedly, practicing nurses do not always see the need for change, and are not always ready for it even when they see the need for it. But to achieve change, there must be genuine commitment.

Success in change implementation requires clearly stated goals, and realistic time frames, as well as empowerment of the people who will participate in the change. We also need adequate staff support, and we need resources. Finally, we need a positive working relationship among the people who are going to implement the change; and that process must be facilitated by consensus decision-making processes (Tagliere, 1992).

Success in change always requires effective leadership. The antithesis of creating change is stifling innovation. The climate of success in change implementation is to constantly test the limits of the people involved, of the process involved, to facilitate in a professional manner, so that we improve the self worth of everybody who is involved in the change.

Transitional and transformational leadership is based on effective communication. Indeed, 100 % of what a leader does is verbal and nonverbal communication. Communication cannot make things worse, and in fact, its objective is to make things better. Remember: there is your truth, and there is my truth, and there is something in between. There are always distortions of the truth when change is about to occur (Kanter, 1989). The leaders who are part of the change process disappear or become a part of the collective when consensus decision-making occurs. (see figure 4).

Figure 4

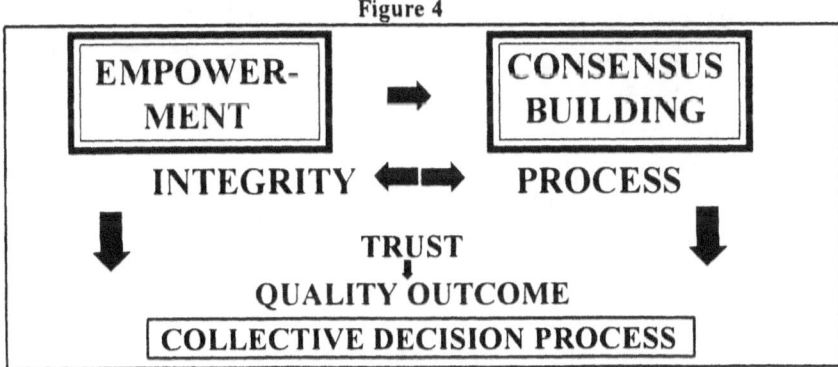

Events and people disappear, or new ones appear to establish conflict resolution, and to be able to achieve consensus on certain issues over time. People change and events change. Over a period of time, whatever truth exists becomes quite a different truth (Kanter, 1983). The essence of implementing change is to remember that no one likes change. No one. But it is our job as nursing leaders to create a change process, and then implement it. So among the critical building blocks of change, is first of all, a willingness to depart from tradition. For those who would say " I'm anxious for the good old days". Let us assure them one and all: the good old days were not as good as they were old.

The second building block is the need for a galvanizing event. The third is strategic decisions that are generated by all those who will be involved with, and affected by the change. These are called the individual prime movers. Kanter calls these people "empowering champions." They make all the difference. They are the leaders in the nursing staff who will solidify individual commitment to the strategy; and they will do it in the informal way that is most effective. They will cultivate other people because they are power sources. This is part of the political process, whether in nursing service, administration, or in nursing education. Whether at the state or federal level, this is an important skill which nurses must learn. The last building block of change is the action vehicle which means making sure that there are mechanisms that will implement the changes that have been decided upon via consensus. These mechanisms make the change possible (Kanter, 1983).

There is nothing worse for a group of nurses who have worked hard in designing a plan than to find they can't put it into action, so the action vehicle is essential. Thus, the promise for resources for implementation are critical. Hospitals in the year 2001 will belong to integrated health care networks, involving:
- off-site emergency room and operating room
- ambulatory surgery
- sub acute services
- alternative treatments
- case management
- outcome benchmarking
- wellness
- fitness
- training and re-training
- telecommunications and the information highway

These changes will involve nursing's growth too. Therefore it is crucial that nurses, at the practice level, be informed of and involved in implementing these changes in our current practice. Nurse leaders involved in strategic planning or strategic development need to be explorers, artists, judges, and warriors. When you are searching for new information, be an explorer. When you are turning your resources into new ideas, be an artist. When you are evaluating the merits of the ideas presented to you, be a judge. And when you are carrying your ideas into action, be a warrior (Van Oech, 1988). Organizations are critical, but nothing replaces leadership. If you are not sure of the changes you want to make, if you are not calm and relaxed about your vision... you may lose the courage of your convictions.

New skills are needed for transformational nursing leaders. The first and most important, is the effective use of power skills and empowering skills: be generous to others, share power. It is amazing how many nurses are fearful of serving on hospital-wide committees, or attending meetings. Sharing your power with them will empower them widely. The second new skill is to manage by consensus, for greater employee satisfaction. The third new skill is understanding how change is designed, recognizing that refreezing is no longer operational; and recognizing that in a revolution new changes occur every single day.

Leadership stimulates individuals to action. Leadership provides service to those who make the money for the hospital. Administration is 100% communication because individuals are important; and they act in response to the expectation of their leaders. If they are not involved, they will not be the stimulator or the receptor of change.

Table 8
PARTICIPATIVE DECISION MAKING PHILOSOPHY

- WE'RE ALL IN THE SAME BOAT
    - -NEED SAME DIRECTION
    - -PATCH THE LEAKS

- APPROPRIATE GOAL - SETTING
    - -NEED TO CONSTANTLY REASSESS

- UNDERLYING COMMITMENT TO INCLUSIVENESS

Leadership requires courage. Courage is fear that has said its prayers. Courage is the quality that guarantees all the other leadership qualities. Ernest Hemingway defined courage as "grace under pressure."

There are two basic rules in life as we reach the end of the 20th century: change is inevitable and everybody resists change. However, leaders who wish to survive into the 21st century will recognize that the transition most essential to this journey is the willingness to empower other nurses at the practice level. Peter Drucker has written that 90 % of the decisions to be made in any organization must be made at the point of service. In nursing this means at the practice level. If you see change as an opportunity, you can see it as an exhilarating, refreshing challenge, even an adventure. Those who work with transformational leaders catch the virus of change.

Change masters are adept at re-orienting their own and others activities into untried directions to bring about ever higher levels of achievement (Kanter, 1989). Change masters encourage new procedures and see new possibilities...this is the development of the vision statement. They encourage the anticipation of, and the response to, external pressures, even in a time of revolution. They listen to new ideas from within...goal setting in what has come to be called the intrapreneur. Transformational leadership characteristics then, for the 21st century involve moving from the old style nursing management to the new style of shared governance or professional nursing practice: (see tables 9, 10, 11)

Table 9

FROM		TO
Directing	→	Facilitating
Controlling	→	Coordinating
Managing	→	Innovating
Doing	→	Delegating
Boss	→	Colleague
Problem finding	→	Problem solving
Directing	→	Coaching

This will allow transformational leaders to assist the nurses at the practice level to shift long standing attitudes in nursing which have not been professionally motivated. Attitude shifts that must occur in the nurse at the practice level can only occur when the transformational leader shows the way (see table 7).

Table 10

FROM		TO
Mistrust	→	Trust
Betrayal	→	Commitment
Blaming Others	→	Working Together
Competitive	→	Cooperative Excellence is the idea
Excellence is Ideal	→	Excellence as Reality
Identity with Group	→	Identity with Fate of Organization

Table 11

21st Century Business Characteristics

- Highly skilled knowledge workers
- Products = knowledge packages
- Global in scope
- Technologically driven
- Rapid change & complexity
- Activities distributed: Time & Space
- Multipurpose and many constituencies
- Fuzzy boundaries

There is no question that in a time of revolution such as the American health care delivery system is in, the critical themes driving change will be to focus primarily on: the mission, the values, and the goals of the American health care delivery system. This must also involve the identity, and the values, and the mission of nursing in the new health care delivery system. All members of the health care delivery system must look at the relationship of health care delivery to the stakeholders. All members in the health care delivery system must look at the way we work, and restructure accordingly. It is important that registered nurses agree on the core values of registered nursing:

1. To achieve success in nursing through client/customer satisfaction
2. To deliver quality service and excellent service in all things
3. To acquire the technology to develop leadership in the health care market
4. To develop and empower nurse employees to their fullest potential
5. Nurses must act as responsible, corporate citizens who are integral to the organization's success

In order for these values to become reality, leaders in a transformational mode, must willingly change the way they manage. Giving up the word "management" would be a good beginning. Leaders... lead. Leaders make site visits to nursing units. Leaders encourage nurses to visit within the organization. Leaders encourage nurses to actively participate in the analysis and evaluation of nursing's care. Nurse leaders organize feedback conferences so that all nurses are involved in the evaluation of nursing's work. (see figure5)

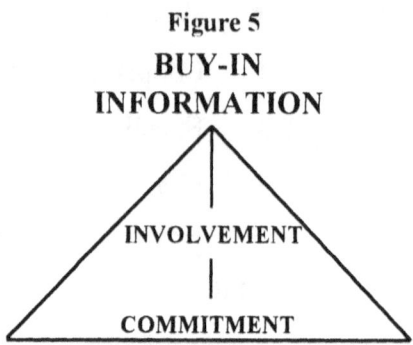

Figure 5
BUY-IN
INFORMATION

INVOLVEMENT

COMMITMENT

It is only when transformational leaders in nursing willingly recognize that a personal involvement on their part is essential to promote organizational awareness among staff nurses, that organizational aversion, in this time of revolution, will be avoided or eliminated. The treatment for organizational aversion, which is rampant in nursing today, is transformational leadership. Transformational leadership is the promotion of the concept by leaders, that everyone in a nursing organization is involved with and affected by the fate of the organization.

Japanese Industry Has A
"SHARED FATE ETHIC*"

*Everyone is involved with and affected by THE FATE of the organization.

Organizational Awareness
vs
Organizational Aversion

Chapter Seven

PLANNING FOR STRATEGIC DEVELOPMENT

Strategic thinking is a way of viewing the organization to be proactive and move the organization toward its desired vision of the future. Strategic thinking involves scanning the internal and external environment of the organization: identifying strengths and weaknesses; threats and opportunities for the delivery of services; and making strategic decisions when key opportunities arise (Bean, 1993).

Strategic planning and strategic development therefore, are processes to develop an organizational plan to attain specific long term goals. This activity is usually done every three to five years. Strategic development follows a needs assessment, and internal analysis, to produce a collaborative process used to define the values, and the culture needed for the nursing department to achieve its vision.

ONE FUTURE SCENARIO:

Welcome to the year 2036. A lot has changed since the old days in nursing, forty years ago, especially throughout the health care field. There is still death, of course, but not from illness; that was taken care of long ago. Technology has made surgery obsolete and you may be surprised to learn that government is picking up most of the health care tab these days. As for hospitals, well, what's a hospital?

This much is certain: almost all of the elements of the health care delivery system that will exist in the mid 21st century are ones which are in embryonic stages today. The two most uncertain elements in predicting what the system of the future will be like are: 1) how far the current vectors for change will extend into the years ahead; and 2) how they will interact in our complex society to produce the health care delivery system demanded for the future of the United States. The one thing we can predict with confidence is that health care has become big business for nurses, physicians, and other health care participants and it will continue to be big business in the year 2036 and beyond. The other thing we can predict with confidence is that health care reform is in its infancy today, and will go on and on well into the next century.

Driving Forces In Health Care Delivery

One conceptual framework on which to base strategic development for a division of nursing consists of ten driving forces that will shape the health care delivery system well into the 21st century (Coile, 1986). The first driving force is aging. By 1990, 12 % of the population of the United States was over the age of 65. That means that by the year 2000, just a few years away, there will be almost six million Americans over the age of 80. The fastest growing segment of the American population is over the age of 80 now.

The second driving force is competition. Competition over the price of health care, and this means that we must find ways so that not only the fiscally fit will survive, but so that 38 million people who are uninsured, and another 30 million people who are underinsured, can also survive and receive health care.

The third driving force is integrated health care systems, which entail extravagant use of home and community resources. The lifeblood of the future will be contracts and discounts. (Contracts with HMOs, contracts with PPOs, contracts with groups of physicians and discounted prices).

The fourth driving force is health care conglomerates. Right now one of every three hospitals in the U.S. is owned by a multi-hospital system. It is predicted that by the year 2000, one out of two will be part of a conglomerate, and 30 % or more of the expenditures for health care will come from business with conglomerates.

The fifth driving force is corporate practice, which means that the practice of medicine in this country is undergoing fundamental change. By the year 2000, nine of ten physicians will no longer be in fee-for-service practice. They will be in group practices and other kinds of hospital partnerships.

The sixth driving force is the new consumer...who is very price conscious. The new consumer will join more HMOs as private insurance companies are eliminated and as health care reform takes hold. There will be lower utilization of health care services. Managed care will become the dominant force in health care reform.

The seventh driving force is information and telecommunications, involving the knowledge explosion regarding health care for the American consumer. The implementation of the information superhighway in health care delivery will guide and direct health care consumerism.

The eighth driving force is the shifting of dollars from inpatient to outpatient services, from fee for service to capitation, and from acute care to long term care. There will be a 50 % reduction in the number of in-hospital patients by the year 2000. It is said that the business of health care by the year 2000 will have shifted to chronic illness and long term care.

The ninth driving force is the bionic age, with increasing use of technology, artificial intelligence, genetic engineering, super drugs, and of course biological replacements for those who can afford them.

The last driving force is shifting values. The issues of life and death will be highly complex, and new bio-ethical issues will be raised. Issues that we haven't even thought about yet will have to be faced tomorrow (Coile, 1986).

Twelve Financial Megatrends
The second framework for strategic planning consists of twelve financial megatrends, which correlate to the preceding driving forces (Coile, 1986).
• The first financial megatrend is from institutionalization to non-institutionalization: fewer people will be admitted to hospitals and those who are admitted will stay for shorter periods of time.
• The second megatrend is from acute to ambulatory care because, as already noted, chronic illness will be the principal business of the health care industry.
• The third is from invasive to noninvasive procedures, which means a 20 % reduction in surgical procedures by the year 2000.
• The fourth financial megatrend is from third party payment to direct contracting, either by the government or by employers, via health care alliances. As a matter of fact, by the year 1984, 80 % of the Fortune 500 companies were already self-insured.
• The fifth financial megatrend is from health insurance to integrated health care systems, because the insurance concept of health care as we have known it is dead, and health care reform mandates managed care.
• The sixth is from insensitive consumer to very price conscious consumer who knows that choice is now determined by who pays the bill.
• The seventh trend is from high margin to low margin pricing.
• The eighth is from local markets to global markets. Globalization will be a key activity of the 21st century.
• The ninth trend is from long term debt to equity capital. We see this already happening in the joint ventures and mergers which are increasing everyday throughout the health care system in this country _(Modern Health Care)._
• The tenth megatrend is from case payment to carload purchase, which means the more people in the managed care plan, the more people in the alliance, the less the plan will cost.

• The eleventh trend is from single product to diversified portfolio. Health care products and services offered by integrated health care systems will be very diverse, a trend that has already begun, but is only the tip of the iceberg thus far.

• The final financial megatrend is from public relations to paid advertising, or what could be called "brand name advertising" for the health care marketplace: tremendous merchandising of health care such as we have never seen before (Coile, 1986).

Strategic Planning

Given these two frameworks, strategic planning is a critical element in the future of every nursing department. It is a tremendous challenge that we must undertake. Strategic planning is defined as the art of formulating beforehand a detailed scheme for accomplishing one or more goals. It is a continuous and systematic process for making risky decisions today with the greatest possible knowledge and awareness of their effect on the future (Bean, 1993).

Five principles of strategic planning are:
1. Critical thinking about the past, the present, and the future;
2. Sensitivity to the needs of the department or the division, its person nel, and its customers;
3. A structured plan that is flexible and adaptable to continuous environ mental change;
4. Accuracy which is increased when outcomes can be measured quantitatively;
5. Advanced planning or proactivity, which is related to making sound decisions for the future in the present time.
(Goodstein, 1992).

In short, strategic planning specifies desired outcomes, maps out the actions to be taken to achieve those outcomes, and then measures the degree of success in outcome achievement. That should sound familiar to those of us in nursing...because we call that: the nursing process.

Strategic planners ask three questions that we must begin to ask as nurses: 1. *Where are we: Assessment.* Assessing strengths, weaknesses, threats, and opportunities. These questions identify the key issues to be studied and it also contains an environmental assessment. 2. *The second question ..* *Where do we want to go?* is the development of a mission statement, and the development of specific strategic goals and objectives that conform to the fulfillment of the mission statement. 3. *The third question... How do we get there?* Is based on actions and plans and an implementation plan to meet the goals and objectives with target dates for completion and individual account-abilities (Nolan, 1993).

Strategic planning is a management activity to help organize and develop increased quality by capitalizing on the strengths we already have. However, as we all know, change is always difficult. It is easy to come up with new ideas. The hard part is letting go of what worked two or three years ago, but will soon be out of date.

Strategic planning for nursing departments deals with: 1) the chang-ing environment in the health care industry; 2) the competitive conditions in the health care industry; 3) the strengths and weaknesses of the department, or unit of nursing; and 4) the opportunities for growth within that depart-ment or division.

In a strategic development process, success is a journey, not a desti-nation.

Leadership

These are indeed " the best of times and the worst of times" for nursing. Most importantly, this is our time of opportunity. And leadership in nursing must change and develop commensurate with that opportunity. Lead-ership in nursing must develop a vision to take us into the year 2000. With-out vision, nursing could die. This new leadership will have to define nursing's retrenchment and redeployment from hospitals to the community... because the community will be the new venue for the practice of nursing.

Finances will be constricted for the rest of our careers. The rapid changes in health care will continue for as long as we practice...and live. The style of today's nursing leader must be active and intrusive. As Will Rogers said, "even if you're on the right track, you'll get run over if you just sit there." The visionary nursing executive today articulates philosophy; makes contact at all levels of the division, and the community; is receptive and expressive; attends to strengths, not weaknesses; and talks about future goals with nursing staff and the community. This means that the great need for anyone in authority in nursing these days is courage. Strategic plan-ning and strategic development require risk-taking. Risk-taking means be-ing willing to make a mistake in an attempt to make progress. Remember, strategic development means being willing to design the future and then make it happen. As Tom Peters (1994) has written, the essence of progress is failure; and action is everything.

Alice in Wonderland said to the Cheshire Cat " Would you please tell me which way I ought to go from here?" and the Cheshire Cat said,

"That depends on where you want to go." This is the most important mission of the nurse leader: to guide and direct the professional staff as a whole in deciding where they want to go. However, innovative policy by its very definition promotes controversy; and nursing leaders will have to expect that, deal with it, and even permit it.

The components of a nursing department are: administration; management; leadership; and staff. Administration means to minister to the needs of those who do the work. The job of a nurse administrator is to see that the professional staff have what they need to do their job. This means attending to a thousand details everyday.

Management asks the question: Do these things really need to be done? Are these things still worth doing? The manager is the navigator through the treacherous channels of constant change for any nursing department. Often the administrator and the manager are the same person.

The third component is leadership, which provides the emotional injections to jolt the staff out of a tendency to coast. This has been called the poetic side of administration. It is the soul of strategic planning and development.

The professional staff must participate, as professionals, in the changing of the profession of nursing, as we move to a new level of practice, meeting new goals and accomplishing new agendas.

To help us with these problems, among the planning activities that we have to undertake is, first: the pursuit of quality. For the administrator this means finding people doing something right; converting those who are "difficult" to your side; turning questions into suggestions. Everybody in nursing management today knows that the better the staff you have in your organization, the better the organization will be. The more empowered the staff are, the more productive they will be.

The second planning activity is information: making sure (before getting into the strategic development mission statement) that we have precise, factual information regarding populations, customers, demography, trends, etc. This kind of information facilitates rational decision making (Goodstein, 1992).

What Is Strategic Planning And Development
Following is a summary of what strategic planning is not: it is not a blueprint; it is not a set of platitudes; it is not vague; and it is not vapid; it is not a personal vision of the administrator; it is not a collection of department plans; it is not a wish list; it is not something done at an annual retreat; it is not a way of eliminating risk, because it actually increases risk; and it is not

an attempt to outwit the future, because it is a set of decisions that the entire nursing department makes in order to secure its future (Goodstein, 1992).

So what is strategic planning? It is being active, not passive, about position in history. It is positive, and it is vigorous, because that's what the word strategic means. It is in step with the changing environment of health care reform, because it looks outward while taking into consideration that three fourths of all change is triggered by outside forces and needs continuous adaptation. This is most certainly true for nursing within the framework of the health care delivery system as it is evolving today. The changes that are needed in nursing are coming from the outside by way of the changes in the health care delivery system itself, and that handwriting is on the wall now (see table 9).

Strategic planning is competitive, because it recognizes economic and market conditions. Strategic planning concentrates on decisions and answers the questions: 1. Where are we? 2. Where do we want to go? 3. How do we get there? 4. What should we do? 5. How shall we decide? 6. Where do we put our energies? (Goodstein, 1992)

Strategic planning is a blend of political maneuvering and psychological interplay...and the process is overt (Nolan, 1993).

Strategic planning is highly participatory, and highly tolerant of controversy. Dissent is permitted, but sabotage is not. So we must establish the ground rules at the beginning of the process. Controversy is probably essential, but sabotage is never tolerated, because strategic planning and development concentrate on the fate of the nursing department above all else (see figures 6, 7).

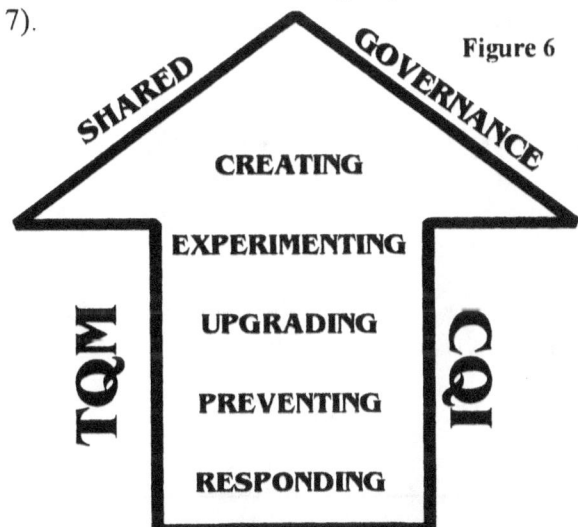

Figure 6

SHARED GOVERNANCE

CREATING

EXPERIMENTING

UPGRADING

PREVENTING

RESPONDING

TQM

CQI

REACTIVE vs PROACTIVE STRATEGIES

Finally, a caveat regarding strategic planning:

A STRATEGIC PLANNING PROCESS

Figure 7

	E
1st PLAN to PLAN	E
STAKEHOLDERS ⬇	V
VALUES ⬇	A
MISSION ⬇	L
VALIDATION WITH COMMUNITIES	U
2nd STRATEGIC DECISIONS ⬇	A
WHAT TO DO	
3rd TACTICAL DECISIONS ⬇	T
HOW TO DO	I
4th ACTION PLANS & IMPLEMENTATION	O
	N

THE PLAN

*In the beginning was the plan. And then came the assump-
tions. And the assumptions were without form. And the plan
was completely without substance, And the darkness was
upon the face of the workers. And they spake unto their
marketing manager, saying, "It is a pot of crap, and it
stinketh." And the marketing manager went unto the strategists and sayeth, "It is a pile of dung, and none may abide
the odor thereof." And the strategists went unto the business managers and sayeth unto them, "It is a container of
excrement, and it is very strong." And the director went
unto the vice president and sayeth, "It contains that which
aids plant growth, and it is very strong." And the vice president went unto the senior vice president and sayeth, "It
promoteth growth, and it is powerful." And the senior vice
president went unto the president and sayeth unto him, "This
powerful new plan will actively promote the growth and
the efficiency of the company and the business in general."
And the president looked upon the plan and saw that it was
good, AND THE PLAN BECAME POLICY.*

- Anonymous

Morale and Moral: Keep the plan dynamic, flexible, a living document !!!

Table 12

STRATEGIC PLANNING - ACTION PLAN

ITEM	ASSESS-MENT #	DUE DATE	ACCOUNT-ABILITY	REAL DATE

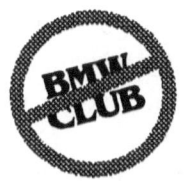

Chapter Eight

THE BMW CLUB

The BMW Club in nursing is something we need to stop, not something we need to join or to earn membership in; but something we must give up. It is the "Bitching, Moaning, and Whining Club." There is a cartoon from Peanuts in which Lucy says, "I suppose you think it's easy being a bitch." Losers say " It may be possible but it's too difficult." Winners say, "It may be difficult, but it's always possible." It is possible and necessary to give up the BMW Club.

In today's society we frequently use the terms "toxic people", and "nourishing people." As you might expect, toxic people/nurses are the ones who always dwell on the negative. Toxic is defined as poisonous; toxic people/nurses continually spread poison. Nourishing is defined as nurturant behavior, or behavior designed to promote growth. People who are nourishing are positive and supportive. They lift our spirits and bring joy to those around them. And that is why we must give up the Bitching, Moaning, and Whining Club. Lucy could be right: it may be difficult. But we must decide...do we wish to be toxic or nourishing nurses?

How do we start giving up the BMW Club? We start by learning how to negotiate. Negotiating means learning how to get all you need, when you can't get all you want. Everyone alive in the health care delivery system in the last ten years either as a purveyor, receiver, or giver of health care, knows we cannot get all we want. That is a given today. How then, can we get all we need?

It has been said that anger is a choice we make when we feel choiceless. When we feel choiceless we become angry. The people with whom we associate have a profound effect on the way we feel, and on the way we ultimately behave. Negative people drag us down to their level. They hammer at us with all the things "you can't do" and all the things they think are impossible. They barrage us with gloomy statements and the problems in life. After listening to toxic people, members of the BMW Club, we feel listless, depressed, and drained.

Life isn't fair, and when compost hits the fan it isn't always evenly distributed. Downbeat attitudes need to be forfeited in order to leave the BMW Club. Negative thinking, or what I am going to call negaholism, is really the underlying cause of all addictive or compulsive behavior. These addictive, compulsive behaviors are usually the result of self imposed pressures to excel in work and in our personal lives. BMW Club members are negaholics.

We all know what alcoholics are, now I present you with negaholics (Carter-Scott, 1991). Negaholics are people who suffer from chronic negativity; and they have out of control negative coping systems. The point is, just the way people who are alcoholics do not admit to being alcoholic, or even recognize their alcoholism, so negaholics oftentimes have no idea that this is their pathology, and their habitual coping behavior. The dominant negative coping behavior for all negaholics is denial. Denial is the strongest mental mechanism or coping mechanism known to man or beast. Just as an alcoholic's first step needs to be admitting to drinking too much, negative copers must acknowledge that they are not fulfilling their potential because pessimism is out of control. Breaking this cycle is essential to maturity. People re-evaluate and begin to see life as a learning adventure, and then they realize that there is no such thing as a negative experience.

The dominant symptom of negaholism is "whinorrhea" (Wooten, 1992). I want to share with you the thought that one way to respond to Lucy whose question is "I suppose you think it's easy being a bitch," by responding, "Lucy, it's not easy being a bitch. You really have to work at it." I am not sure we even realize the energy it takes to be that kind of negative. It is true that we in nursing are continually faced by great opportunities brilliantly disguised as unsolvable problems. Surely that can make us suffer from negaholism, this terrible disease of chronic negative coping.

However, the truth is that negaholism is a contagious, corporate syndrome (Carter-Scott, 1991). Anyone who works in a hospital setting works in a corporate environment. So negaholism is a contagious, corporate syndrome, endemic in nurses who are employed in hospitals.

This contagious, corporate syndrome results in three things that the nursing profession has suffered from throughout my career. First of all: mediocrity. Secondly: complacency. And thirdly: infighting. These are the results of membership in the BMW Club.

Negaholics limit their own innate abilities. They are responsible for their own limitations. They convince themselves that they can never be happy in their work...and they are not. That is their business: to convince themselves that no job will ever make them happy, because they can never get what they want. And finally because of these limitations, and negative self talk, they sabotage their own dreams; and because they cannot stand to be sabotaged alone...they sabotage us too. Personal negativity frequently results from dysfunctions which we sustain in our childhood; and do not wish to address in a therapeutic environment. Some nurses are fed-up with hearing about co-dependency. Personally I am not. I am co-dependent; and it helps me to remember that when I talk about it, when I read about it, or when I talk to myself about it. If women in the American society tend to be co-dependent (and in my opinion, we do) it takes willful, personal, self-growth, in a therapeutic environment, to get over the habit of personal negativity. Personal negativity comes from the dysfunctions of childhood and leads straight into the work environment, where it is rarely identified and rarely treated (Larson and Goodstein, 1993).

William James, one of our greatest and earliest American psychologists, wrote that the greatest discovery of his generation of psychotherapists was that human beings alter their lives by altering their attitudes. When nurses think about the vast influence of attitudinal change and attitudinal shifting that can occur when nurses leave the BMW Club, the extensions are mind boggling. Our behavior affects not only our work, but our homes, our families and our friends.

The clues of negaholism are those which deal directly with "I can't," "they won't", and "I am not able." Additionally, clues to negaholism abound in nursing because nurses suffer from nurse abuse. Frequently the perpetrators of nurse abuse are other nurses. If you have experienced that, you need to address how to cure what Gasparis and Swirsky (1990) have called horizontal violence (not vertical violence), because it is not the vice president of nursing or the CEO dumping on us. It is us, dumping on each other...and that is a result of the BMW Club. Negativity is habituating. We do not even hear ourselves when we do it; and the receiver accepts it as if it were normal behavior.

There are four categories of negaholism: attitudinal; behavioral; mental; and verbal negaholism (Carter-Scott, 1991). *The attitudinal negaholic* is the negaholic who is always deeply dissatisfied. This is the negaholic

39

nurse about whom we say in our work setting, "Oh, don't pay any attention, that's just the way s/he is." But we do pay a lot of attention because negaholism is a contagious, corporate syndrome. It is a communicable disease. If it is contagious, we catch it. Attitudinal negaholics are horrific. They frequently are workaholics. If you need something done in a hurry give it to an attitudinal negaholic. That's the good news. The bad news is they do work hard, but bitch, moan, and whine about it. And they are not team players. So these are workaholic nurses who love control.

Did you ever meet a nurse who did not love control? I do not know whether we became nurses because we love control, or if we became control freaks because we became nurses. It is necessary to remember that nurses are very controlling people. Remember, attitudes are deep rooted feelings and beliefs. Therefore, attitudinal negaholics have deep seated negative feelings and beliefs about themselves, their work, and their world.

The behavioral negaholic is personally destructive by "acting out." You see the negative behavior. They are back stabbers, and saboteurs. They want to maintain the status quo, so they are status quo sustainers. They are change resisters, and they work to fulfill self-fulfilling prophecies, with their negative coping behaviors.

The mental negaholic is a constant self-flogger. This nurse always sees the glass as half empty. It all goes on in the mind. It is not acting out, therefore it is not behavioral, it is all "head stuff." The very eccentric suffer from tremendous mood swings and melancholia. As co-dependents, we would do anything to make this nurse feel better, when in fact we need to understand that this nurse is never going to feel better, unless s/he voluntarily gets into recovery. They are the walking wounded of nursing's world. Their negative coping is all in their heads, and they never see themselves as able to be happy. Therefore, they are constantly self-flogging, using negative self-talk to maintain their membership in the BMW Club.

The verbal negaholic sends negative messages without even knowing that s/he is saying negative things...that is how habitual it is. They love gossip, and they love innuendo. In fact, rumor and innuendo are the lifeblood of the verbal negaholic. They are hypercritical, and they are cynical, not just skeptical. They say things like, "It doesn't matter, why bother, they'll never let us do it, all this stuff is just for show, none of it is for dough"-all the negatives you have heard so often. Here again we have the self-fulfilling prophecy. The verbal negaholic says "Things will never change"; and the verbal and the behavioral negaholics make very sure they do not change by maintaining the status quo.

Negaholics have a great fear of abandonment. This comes from childhood long before nursing school. Negaholics focus on a need to exert excessive control in order to feel comfortable. All nurses, probably all people, have unresolved control issues.

Negaholics have problems with boundaries. They do not like porous boundaries. They like very clearly defined boundaries. They also have problems with reality...they deny reality often. Things have changed in health care since 1983: everything that was offered before 1983 is ancient history and we live in a boundary-less society. The reality in nursing today is that we do not have to do anything the way we did it before 1983. But negaholics in their pathology, simply do not like change of any kind. Negaholics have problems with responsibility as well as irresponsibility. They consider irresponsible behavior anything that does not fit into their personal guidelines of responsible behavior. How many times have you heard nurses on a unit say, "I don't know why she's going to school, a master's degree isn't going to do anything for her." Or how many times have you heard nurses "pull up the ladder" after themselves as in, "I got a baccalaureate degree but no one else needs one." That is negaholism!

When I was going through that nonsense on my trip up the career ladder in nursing I never had the courage, or even the good sense, to say to that nurse who was trying to scare me, "How did you make it?" But for all those who are on the fast track, and wanting to know how to get ahead today, I will tell you that your advanced degrees are tickets, in the most positive sense. They are the most positive tickets for eliminating horizontal violence that I know of; and they assist us in leaving the BMW Club by strengthening our own self confidence, and our own sense of self worth.

Negaholics love to be liked. They have a great need to be liked, but they are not aware of the fact that they drive people away by their abusive communication and behavior. If you ask, "Do you like to be liked?" they will say, "Yes, and I'm very well loved." But the truth lies elsewhere. Negaholics are pushers, not movers and shakers. Negaholics have tremendous needs for drama and chaos. If there is not enough drama and chaos within the system, they will make some. And they have great difficulty with loyalties. These are not loyal nurses, unless their loyalty is to another negaholic person.

Negaholics have problems with guilt. Erma Bombeck has said that guilt is the gift that keeps on giving. But guilt can provide energy for positive change.

It is very easy to merge back with the negaholic virus. Relapse is a constant concern. Since this is a very virulent, contagious virus, it is very easy to have a relapse. If you are really interested in getting out of the BMW

Club and giving up negaholism, you need to get into recovery.

Without any sense of false pride, I willingly admit that I am a recovering negaholic. The secret to my staying in recovery is being surrounded by enough cooperative people, who are either already in recovery, or are eager to get into recovery, so that together we assist each other in maintaining that recovery.

Finally, to maintain my recovery I have to accept the "loyalty challenge" which makes me agree to not do everything myself. My personal recovery is maintained by my agreeing that if nurses have made a commitment with their visions and their values, I am going to have faith and trust in those who are going to accomplish these goals and objectives with me. In other words, my recovery from negaholism is based on the same program that alcoholic recovery is based on. I agree not to do everything myself and thereby give up some of my own unresolved control issues:

I Can Do Something.
I am but one, but I am one.
I cannot do everything, but I can do something.
What I can do I ought to do and what I ought to do with God's help, I will do.

-Anonymous

Another issue in maintaining my personal recovery is understanding that confrontation is letting you know what I see, what I hear, and what I feel; so that you can choose whether or not you want to do something about it. Nurses are very weak in confrontation. Most of us would rather die (or remain negaholic) than confront another nurse, because we all think of confrontation as a defensive, angry stand. It is not.

In order to maintain my recovery from negaholism I either have to talk it out, or I will act it out (as a member of the BMW Club). We need tutoring in the art of confrontation. We need to be coached in the art form of confrontation so we do not sabotage.

We must find new pathways for our own personal growth. Recovery is just the beginning. The first and most important treatment of negaholism is identification of how you tolerate it, in yourself and in others. Identify how you handle negaholism in yourself and then confront others by saying, for example, "I really don't want to be this kind of negative and I want you to help me." Say it to the most negative person on your unit: "Mary, I've gotten into the habit of tremendous negaholism, and I want to change this, and I want you to help me. And by the way, Mary, I'll help you too, and the rewards for both of us will be enormous." Please remember dear colleague, that self-esteem is simply the reputation you have with yourself.

Recovery is just the beginning, because maintaining recovery requires a great commitment. Being committed to seeing it through to a real change in attitude, behavior and self-talk.

Here are some steps you can take to maintain your recovery:
1) If you regularly have lunch with toxic-negaholic people at work, stop having lunch with these people. Extricate yourself from these venomous and poisonous colleagues. 2) If you have a negaholic relative, it is important to put some limits on your involvement with h/her. You need to limit your time, and your energy because negaholism is a very contagious condition. And it is easy to merge back with the negaholic virus. 3) Join business groups or church groups or community organizations which have members who share your values, your goals, and your positive attitude. Become a *posa-holic*. 4) You can also form your own group, with other nursing colleagues or friends who are interested in getting into recovery, and maintaining recovery from negaholism. Your group can be small or it can be large; but it must contain people who are willing to meet on a regular basis and maintain their commitment to behavioral change and attitude shifting.

Let us all move from the BMW Club to the *Lexus* Association.

Lexus stands for:	Loving
	Empathic
	Xenophilic
	&
	Utterly
	Serene

Joining the *Lexus* Association will indicate very clearly to each of us that we have moved from the juvenile status of club membership to the professional status of association members. As *posaholics* who are members of the Lexus Association, we are ready to maintain our recovery. Nurses know that commitment involves a lot of boredom and sometimes anger. It is not a peak experience every hour of every day. Listening actively to everyone (including ourselves) means responding appropriately. We must take each of these situations very seriously. You are an owner in this proposition. Focus on problem-seeking and problem-solving...not on the problem.

> Be careful of the words you say, Keep them soft and sweet. You never know from day to day, Which ones you'll have to eat. *Anonymous*

You cannot change the world. You cannot change others. But you do have the ability to change yourself. And in changing yourself, you can have a very positive impact.

Two things that help me remain a negaholic in recovery (even though there are relapses): first, is the very simple prayer, "God bless those who care enough to object to the BMW Club, and who care enough to object to every kind of negaholism". Second, is this parable:

> Consider the walnut. If you compare the walnut with some of the beautiful and exciting things which grow on our planet, it does not seem to be a marvelous creation. It is common, rough, not particularly attractive and certainly not valuable in any monetary sense. Of course, this is the wrong way to judge a walnut. Break one open and look inside and see how the walnut has grown to fill every nook and cranny available to it. It had no say in the size or shape of that shell but given those limitations, it achieved its full potential for growth. How lucky we will be if like the walnut, we are found to blossom and bloom in every crevice of the professional life that has been given to us. And so my dear nursing colleagues, take heart, for if one nut can do it so can we all. *Anonymous*

We live in the most demanding times of predictable uncertainty that our country has ever seen. These are very hazardous times for all citizens of the United States; and it is hazardous for those of us who grew up in nursing within a heritage of punishment. We must shrug off the bonds of our heredity and our environment. We cannot direct the winds...but we can adjust our own sails!!

Table 13

REMEMBER:
• Blaming is not changing
• Give up the magical wish
• Labeling can help
• Understanding can help
• Leverage is in the interaction
• Timing is everything
• Coping is a daily effort and change is never easy

Chapter Nine

EMPOWERMENT

"All this high falutin "stuff" about running companies boils down to - SURPRISE - the folks who actually do the work." Tom Peters

TRUE EMPOWERMENT =

Responsibility + Authority +
Accountability =

OWNERSHIP

Traditional organizational structures are often depicted as trees. The reason why, is that parts can be dead for years before they drop off; they shelter some and block out the sun for others; anything that drops from the top reaches the bottom quickly and the middle branches bend with ease; from the very top one can see for miles in all directions, except vertically downward; and monkeys can get to the top with remarkable speed. No wonder traditional bureaucratic nursing structures are dysfunctional and dis-empowering. Is it any wonder that we who are in nursing as we reach the end of the 20th century feel that yesterday is a dream, tomorrow is a vision, and today is a bitch? The truth is that excellence can be attained if we care more than others think is wise...if we wish more than others think is safe...if we dream more than others think is practical...and if we expect more than others think is possible. Even then, reality insists that health care is in a revolution and peace is nowhere in sight.

I grew up believing that the autocratic manager in nursing was the norm. During my developmental years in nursing, the autocratic manager behaved in the following ways: 1) she said little unless something was wrong; 2) usually was not interested in the ideas of other nurses; 3) decided what information the staff nurses needed; 4) changed demands unexpectedly; 5) was difficult to talk to; 6) discouraged us from taking risks; 7) set objectives for all subordinates; 8) personally determined performance standards for appraisal.

Today we are eager to promote empowerment and professional development on the part of all participants as a primary part of the leadership role in nursing. The developmental or transformational leader/manager believes that nurses enjoy their work, and can direct, and can control them-

45

selves within the work setting. They recognize that nurses accept and seek responsibility for their own actions. (see table 14 and figure 8)

Table 14

Characteristics of the developmental-transformational leader/manager are:
1) considers ideas that are conflictive with his own
2) allows for a reasonable margin of error
3) helps others learn from mistakes while respecting risk taking
4) consistently expects high performance
5) encourages staff nurses to reach in new directions
6) helps the staff nurse understand objectives and roles of their jobs
7) allows staff nurses to make their own commitments
8) sets objectives with staff nurses for determination of performance appraisal (Adapted from Bethel, 1990).

Figure 8

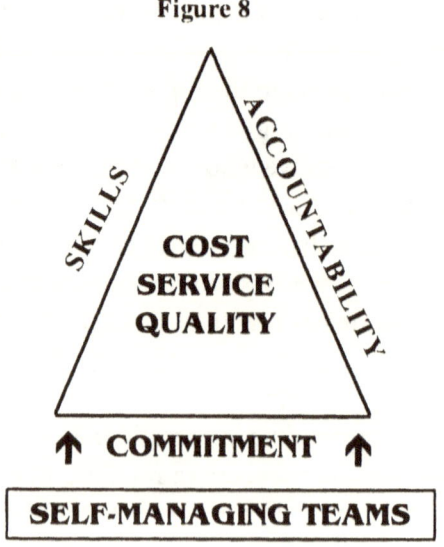

To further delineate the old versus the new manager/leader in nursing here are some words that describe the *old type autocratic nurse leader:*

- **Domineering**   • **Manipulating**
- **Intimidating**   • **Competitive**
- **Harsh**   • **Critical**
- **Decisive**   • **Direct**

Here are words typically used to describe the *empowering transformational leader/manager* who is focused on the development of self managing teams in nursing:

- **supportive**
- **analytical**
- **stable**
- **assured**
- **planner**
- **agile**
- **flexible**
- **understanding**
- **confident**
- **trusting**
- **approachable**
- **tolerant**

A paradigm is a model or structure. Attitude is important in any paradigm shift. Paradigms themselves become theoretical frameworks that can be seen as the final solution. A paradigm can also be the death of anything really happening, because nothing can change without attitudes shifting. The right match between attitude and paradigm is essential. The manager/leader's priorities must change; the staff nurses' priorities must change; and both manager/leaders and staff nurses must recognize that "one size fits all" management or leadership simply doesn't succeed anymore. John Naisbitt and Patricia Aburdene (1992) have written that the major problem of the 90s and beyond is not the re-training of workers, it is the *re-training* of management.

Therefore, as involves nursing and nurses, leading the staff who manage the care is critical, if paradigms and attitudes are to shift to accommodate to health care reform as it will continue in the 21st century. (see figures 9 & 10)

Figure 9

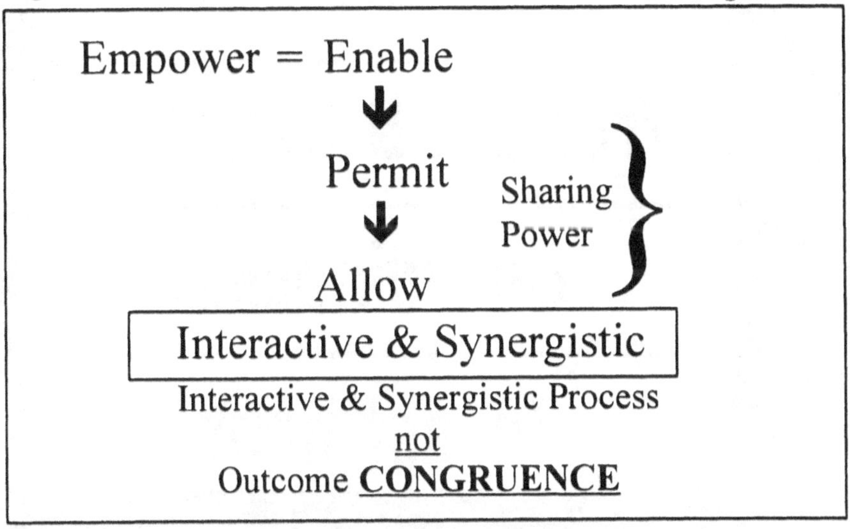

Empower = Enable
↓
Permit   Sharing
↓   Power   }
Allow

| Interactive & Synergistic |

Interactive & Synergistic Process
<u>not</u>
Outcome **CONGRUENCE**

Figure 10

EMPOWERMENT
PRINCIPLES
Congruence
Interdependence
Excellence
Integration
Process & Direction
Coordination
Investment

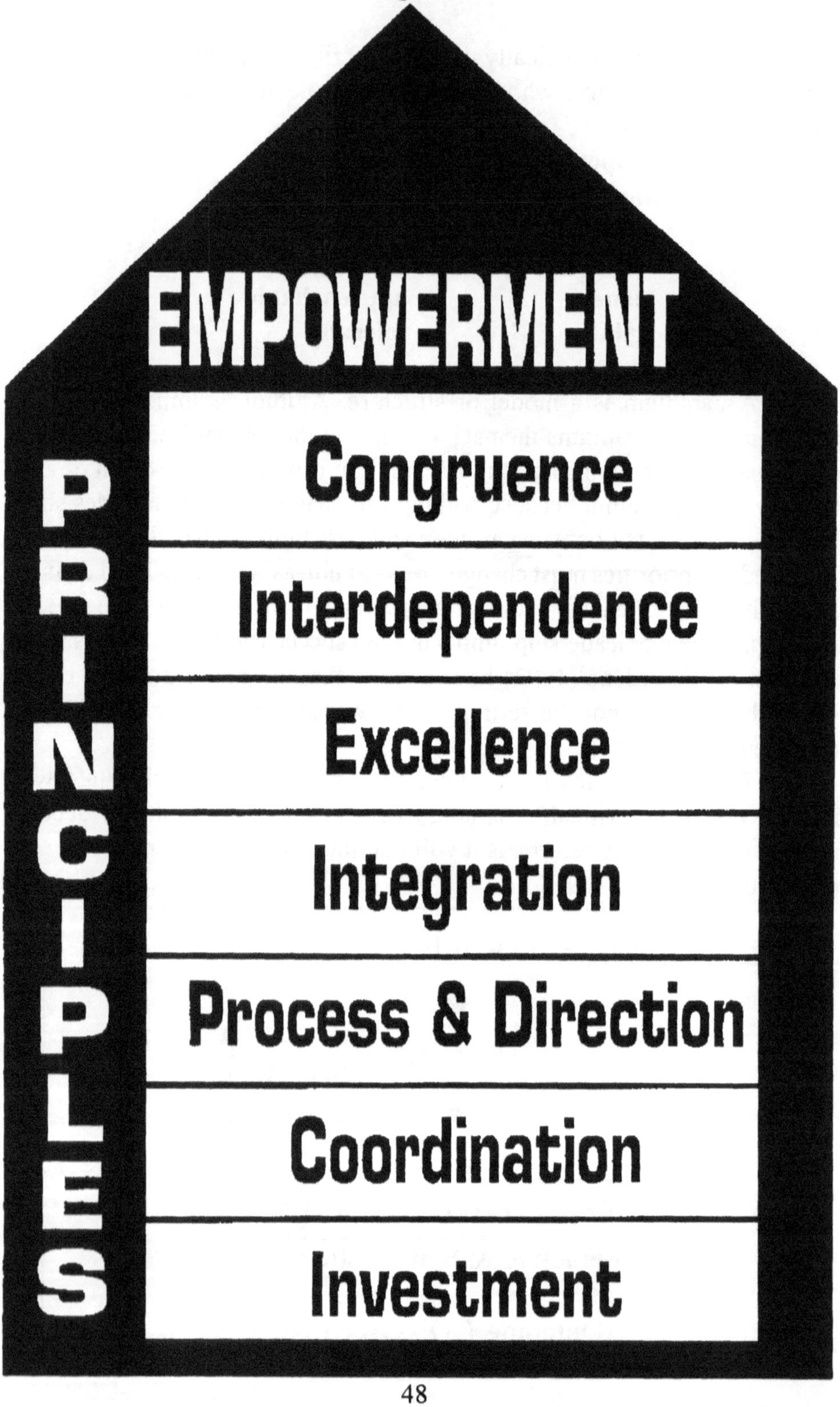

Further, one can say that 90 % of the decisions being made in hospitals today need to be made at the point of service. Put another way, this means that nurses must be empowered to make decisions at the point of service to meet customers' needs. This is congruent with continuous quality improvement, with the principles of empowerment, with the elimination of negaholism, and the promotion of risk taking and confidence-building in professional nurses. Fulton Ousler wrote that we (as human beings) place ourselves between two thieves: regret for yesterday and fear of tomorrow. This is especially true, in my view, of registered nurses.

The essence of management in the 90s and beyond is to give power to registered nurses to strengthen them so that they too can give up regret for yesterday; and fear of tomorrow. Giving registered nurses important work to do on critical issues, giving registered nurses discretion and autonomy over the tasks and resources they know best, giving visibility to registered nurses and providing them with recognition for their efforts...these are the critical factors in empowering leadership today.

Vision is the foundation for the essence of survival in health care today; but vision must be derived form the people, who will have to implement it. The staff nurse needs to incorporate the vision statement within h/her practice and make it a living, breathing thing. When constructed by those who will implement it at the bedside, vision will help us organize thoughts and actions in nursing practice, guide our decision making in nursing practice, clarify problems and define issues in nursing practice, and help in the achievement of organizational re-design and re-alignment and re-structuring.

Figure 11
Nursing's Vision Statement

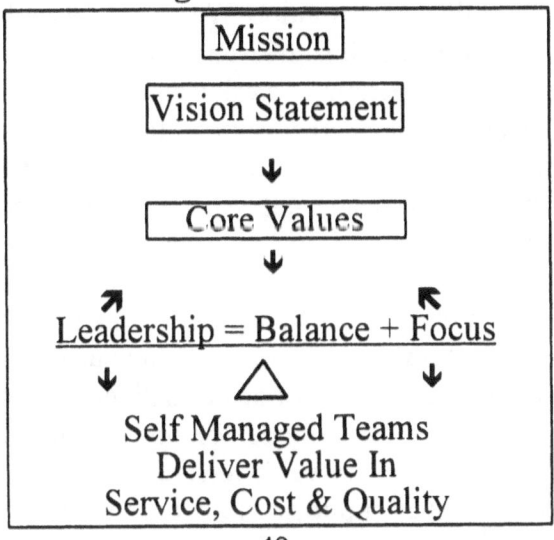

49

A vision also helps to maintain a sense of continuity, while setting the appropriate tone for the organization in which nursing is practiced. We must become continuously customer driven, recognizing that everything we do has the patient/customer in mind. That must be the driving force of the nursing department's vision.

The vision statement has to be very clear, because there are hard decisions ahead of all of us in health care reform for the foreseeable future. I know of no one in health care, including Bill Clinton, who's ready to say right now exactly what form health care reform will take. We know that this process will evolve well into the next century. What we do know is that there will be incremental changes over a substantial period of time. Some of those changes may be small, some of larger magnitude; but over the next seven to eight years we know there will be constant change.

This will be so irrespective of who is President of the United States. Health care reform is on a track that will not be stopped. For the empowering nurse leader at all levels, your career will be limitless.

We've heard for years that people in America change their careers at least four times during their lifetime. This has not been true of nurses until recently. Nurses will not be leaving nursing, but they will be changing their practice setting frequently within the profession. Developing a vision statement, both personal and professional, must be done by including all constituencies; and the guiding words must be transformational... accommodating to incremental change.

George Bernard Shaw wrote: "The people who get on in this world, are those who get up and look for the circumstances they want, and, if they can't find them, make them." This is an especially important message for leaders of nurses in a time of revolution. We are in a period of great experimentation, requiring some caution, great analysis, and high risk taking. This is not the time to be an autocratic or weak leader of nurses. Nurses need to know that their leader will be there to support them as they implement new kinds of nursing service, new kinds of management, and new attitudes.

The transformational leadership skills of empowerment, shared governance, consensus decision-making, and strategic planning, all involve developing, but not controlling and not directing. Professional nurses are able to control and direct and certainly manage their own practice.

The power must reside with the practicing nurse. These are the core values of shared governance and of transformational, empowering leadership within a professional practice model. Empowerment is the core of leadership in professional practice. Nevertheless, for anyone in management today, there is a price to pay. Political skills are the art of influence. Any leader who does not learn to influence will, in my view, fail too many times. Politics is the art of what is possible, and political skill is the art of influencing what is possible to actually happen.

Registered nurses who are empowered will have to learn political skill. Political skills are roughly divided into the following activities: 1) proactively seeking opportunities to provide for the comfort of subordinates because you care about them; 2) continually reevaluating priorities because in a revolution priorities may change everyday; 3) openness to change because the only thing we can count on is predictable uncertainty; 4) being adept at selling others on the concepts of registered nursing and the importance of registered nursing; 5) avoiding reliance upon unchallenged authority... because there is no unchallenged authority in a revolution or in the new world of nursing. The goal therefore becomes one of developing self-managing teams of nurses which are very comfortable in sharing power and using political skill (see figure 8 in this chapter).

WHY EMPOWERMENT??
1. Recognizing that your survival is in your own hands
2. Having a clear sense of purpose
3. Having a commitment to a purpose

In assessing our own empowering leadership skills, we can ask ourselves these questions: 1) Do I encourage the participation of others; 2) Do I set realistic goals; 3) Do I question myself; 4) Do I use group dynamics and facilitation skills to increase loyalty; 5) Do I become a part of the group before initiating action; 6) Do I compete fairly within the system in which I work; 7) Do I have a high frustration tolerance; 8) Do I accept winning without gloating; 9) Can I lose without pouting; 10) Can I control the impulse to get even; 11) Do I willingly share applause with those who do the work?

Empowering leaders eagerly pursue ways to improve teamwork. They recognize that self-managing teams are totally possible in nursing, although they are not common at this time. Registered professional nurses are able to be self-managing once their leaders have instilled this desire, and this confidence in them. Here are six ways to improve teamwork:

Table 15

SIX WAYS TO IMPROVE TEAMWORK ACTION CHECKPOINT

ACTION	CHECKPOINT
1) Stress team goals	1) Clarify and repeat goals as often as necessary
2) Let nurses develop goals	2) Achieve agreement on goals from team members
3) Stress cooperation among team members	3) Diagnose reasons for team members lack of success and encourage cooperation
4) Show nurses how they can help each other	4) Provide support via specifically rewards for team success
5) Emphasize individual contributions to team efforts	5) Identify reasons for failed assignments
6) Treat each nurse as a valued member of the team	6) Listen! Seek! Applaud!!!

The transformational, empowering leader needs to be aware of the following *absolute ways to fail* during this revolution of health care reform: 1) refuse to share your power; 2) organize the opposition; 3) be arrogant; 4) disregard the feelings of staff nurses; 5) defer to upper level management; 6) take big financial risks without just cause; 7) ignore your competition; 8) refuse to empower the professional nursing staff; 9) refuse to coach the professional nursing staff; 10) refuse to take risks of any kind.

Finding the pathway to commitment and empowerment in nursing is essential if nursing as a profession is to survive, and even thrive in the 21st century. Remember that the focus for the journey for health care reform will last for many years: it is a process not just a destination. We must, as professional nurses, develop ties that bind within our profession and within our individual organizations. Ties that bind will spell success. I will close this chapter by sharing with you something that I hope will illustrate better than my words can what empowerment feels like. This is taken from the work of Antoine St. Exupery's The Little Prince:

It was then that the fox appeared.

"Good morning," said the fox.

"Good morning," the little prince responded politely, although when he turned around he saw nothing.

"I am right here," the voice said, "under the appletree."

"Who are you?" asked the little prince, and added, "You are very pretty to look at."

"I am a fox," the fox said.

"Come and play with me," proposed the little prince. "I am so unhappy."

"I cannot play with you," the fox said. "I am not tamed."

"Ah, please excuse me," said the little prince.

But, after some thought, he added:

"What does that mean—'tame'?"

"It is an act too often neglected," said the fox.

"It means to establish ties."

"'To establish ties'?"

"Just that", said the fox.

"But if you tame me, then we shall need each other. To me, you will be unique in all the world. To you, I shall be unique in all the world."

"I am beginning to understand," said the little prince. "There is a flower... I think that she has tamed me."

"It is possible," said the fox. "On the Earth one sees all sorts of things."

"Oh, but this is not the Earth!" said the little prince.

The fox seemed perplexed, and very curious.

"On another planet?"

"Yes."

"Are there hunters on that planet?"

"No. Ah, that is interesting! Are there chickens?"

"No. Nothing is perfect," sighed the fox. The fox gazed at the little prince, for a long time. "Please — tame me!"

"I want to, very much," the little prince replied. "But I have not much time. I have friends to discover, and a great many things to understand."

"One only understands the things that one tames," said the fox. "If you want a friend, tame me."

"What must I do, to tame you!" asked the little prince. "One must observe the proper rites."

"What is a rite?" asked the little prince.

"Those are actions too often neglected," said the fox. So the little prince tamed the fox. And when the hour of his departure drew near -

"Ah," said the fox. "I shall cry."

"It is your own fault," said the little prince. "I never wished you any sort of harm; But you wanted to tame me."

"That is so," said the fox.

"Then it has done you no good at all!"

"It has done me good," said the fox. "Go and look again at the roses. You will understand now that yours is unique in all the world. Then come back to say goodbye to me, and I will make you a present of a secret."

And he went back to meet the fox.

"Goodbye," he said.

"Goodbye," said the fox. "And now here is my secret...a very simple secret: It is only with the heart that one can see rightly; what is essential is invisible to the eye."

"What is essential is invisible to the eye," the little prince repeated, so that he would not forget.

"Men have forgotten this truth," said the fox. "But you must not forget it. You become responsible, forever, for what you have tamed."

That is the essence of empowerment: to change power relationships in nursing. Using transformational leadership, we will "tame" each other and gain mutuality of purpose, vision, hope and process.

Chapter Ten
LEADING IN THE NEW AGE OF NURSING

"For fragmentation is now very widespread, not only throughout so ciety, but also in each individual; and this is leading to a kind of gen eral confusion of the mind, which creates an endless series of problems and interferes with our clarity of perception so seriously as to prevent us from being able to solve most of them. The notion that all these frag ments are separately existent is evidently an illusion, and this illusion cannot do other than lead to endless conflict and confusion" Bohm (1980).

Marilyn Fergueson, a well-respected health science writer, has written the following: "It's not so much that we're afraid of change or so in love with the old ways, but it's that place in between that we fear...it's like being between trapezes. It's like Linus is when his blanket is in the dryer. There's nothing to hold on to." Times are hard in health care and for nurses. People in the American society as, well as nurses, are consumed by crisis and frag-mentation. The challenges posed at this end point of the 20th century are unprecedented. As nurses and as persons of the American society, we are being bombarded by change...omnipresent and accelerating. The society in which we live is in a time of major disruptive force. Nurse leaders must be willing to continue the radical experiment of re-structuring, re-making, and re-designing nursing so that the remainder of the `90s fulfills the prophesy of this decade of the nurse. The decade of the nurse must be surrounded by vast changes in both nursing education and nursing practice. Those changes both in curriculum and in practice must be epitomized by the following characteristics:

1) the nurse as a master designer of quality in health care
2) the nurse as primary contributor in the development of commu nity health centers and the prevention of disease
3) the nurse at the center of patient centered care
4) the nurse as the central concept in promoting a healing environ ment with alternative methods of healing
5) the nurse as micromanager of cost reduction in health care deliv ery
6) the nurse as care giver finally recognized as central to the new health care delivery system
7) the nurse as essential to maintaining momentum in the health care revolution (Modern Healthcare & The American Nurse 1992, 1993, 1994).

In the minds of many in the United States, including senators and congress persons, the United States is presently witnessing its largest business/industry re-organization ever. In health care, this will result in the development of integrated health care systems, the like of which we have never seen before.

The four distinguishing attributes of the future health care system will be: 1) vertical integration: whereby payors contract with one party for a broad spectrum of care (doctors and hospitals sign as one party); 2) geographic coverage: moving away from small community hospital orientation as a service area, and moving toward regionalization of health care delivery; 3) capitation: provider systems assume risk for the whole of the patient's care; coverage is for life e.g., "whatever is required"; 4) low cost and total care for "covered lives" provided at the lowest possible cost. Integrated health care systems enable much care to be delivered in clinics and in homes with hospital utilization very slender.

These integrated health care systems will be characterized by: 1) a strong customer orientation; 2) a community orientation; 3) high quality; low cost care; 4) serving specific populations; 5) effective hospital physician relationships; 6) effective physician leadership; 7) innovative financing e.g., hospital/physician associations and partnerships.

The movement towards universal coverage, requires leaders in nursing to recognize these differences. Today we must look for nurses who are creative, and who are able to color outside the lines they were trained and/or educated for initially. For those of us who were educated or trained in the "good old days", this means doing and thinking in ways we were not prepared for in our nursing programs.

The future leaders of nursing must be developed by us, the present leadership in nursing. We must assist them to understand that the new health care environment's success will be based on: 1) achievement of outcomes; 2) financial integrity of the integrated health care system; 3) adaptation to change of physician staff, nursing staff, and administration; 4) flexibility and agility in response to change; 5) productivity (do more with less but do it better) 6) cost control; 7) high quality service that satisfies the customer and the family; 8) quality...quality...quality...according to the customer's definition.

The nurse working in the hospital setting would answer "Yeah!" to the pronouncement: "You are either overworked or unemployed in hospital nursing today." There is no question that the organizations of health care delivery are more demanding than they have ever been before, and are likely to remain so. Nevertheless, the future of nursing's leadership lies in recognizing that *90 % of the decisions made in hospitals should be made by the nurse at the practice level, who meets the customer's needs.* Nurses in hospital settings today are very concerned about their futures; and are in greater need of leadership support than ever before.

Hospitals across this country are re-engineering. They are asking the question "If we crashed and had to rebuild what should we keep? How should we do it? And who, in fact, should do it" (Hammer & Champy, 1993). In nursing this is called work re-structuring or work re-design or even patient focused care. It is simply the analysis of the work being done today in hospitals so that nurses can make appropriate decisions in terms of service, quality and cost. The questions nurse leaders must ask are: What is being done? Who is doing it? Should it be done? And if it should be done, who is the best person (for service, cost, quality) to do it ?

These are very scary questions for the nurse at the practice level. The answers to these questions, and more importantly, the implementation of the answers to these questions, require enormous skill and confidence on the part of the leader implementing work re-design in any hospital today.

The major reason for this change relates to the salary increases of the registered nurses in the hospital setting over the last ten years. Realistically, there are going to be fewer nurses working in hospitals in the future. The dominant domain for the registered nurse in the future is the community. The hospital nurse will be heavily supported with the utilization of unlicensed assistive personnel (UAP).

The UAPs will do the tasks that are not cost effective for registered nurses to perform and which do not require that level of expertise. The leader's job will be to assist registered nurses at the practice level to make appropriate decisions regarding delegation and accountability within the legal, moral, and ethical domains of nursing's practice. Leadership's job therefore is to remove obstacles so the registered nurse and the UAP can do their jobs in an efficient, quality focused manner. As a diploma trained nurse I grew up with the following rules:

- Don't rock the boat.
- Don't enjoy your work.
- Don't disagree with the boss.
- Don't volunteer.
- Look busy even when you're not.
- Don't be associated with failures.
- Don't take risks.
- Don't be the bearer of bad news.
- Don't share information with others.
- And complain, complain, complain.

These were the good old days!?!

However, as we approach the 21st century the great need for inspirational leadership, and the great need for empowerment have changed those rules. The nurse leader of today knows that s/he must:
- Treat all workers with respect.
- Enjoy your work and assist others to enjoy their work.
- Encourage nurses to have fun at work.
- Speak with pride about the organization and expect others to do likewise.
- Initiate changes and promote flexibility.
- Be a risk taker.
- Be first, Be focused, Be fit.
- Bring uncomfortable issues into the open.

The expectations for the health care business and how it will be run in the 21st century is that the health care environment will flourish where trust flourishes and is characterized by:
- Integrity
- Respect
- Empowerment
- Vision
- Communications
- Sacrifice
- Small budgets
- Conflict resolution
- Recognition, authority and accountability

The vision of nursing in the future, is very attractive, inspiring, even compelling. Securing this new future in the 21st century means that we as leaders in nursing must take up the characteristics of the new community of business. We are willing to be proactive business persons in moving the health care delivery system to a community based integrated health care system. We recognize that the world in which we live and work will be smaller, environmentally safe, and economically limited. This means needing to change our values, our beliefs and even our philosophies (Maynard & Mehrtens, 1993).

It means recognizing: 1) that relationships will be dependent on connectedness; 2) that authority will be the antithesis of competition; 3) that values will mean decreasing our love of materialism and increasing our spirit of inner trust and security; 4) recognizing that the mode of inquiry in the 21st century will change from linear to intuitive, and that decision making will be characterized by consensus (Barrentine, 1993).

We will tap into a full range of human cognitive and perceptual abilities that have not been usual business characteristics. Many of us are not even aware of these characteristics. And yet they will be nursing's strength in the next century as the entire society places caring in health care as a useful parameter of continuous quality improvement (Galbraith, 1993).

The proactive, ultrapreneur nurse leader of the 21st century will value relationships above all else, and will understand that it makes more sense to shape the future than to fight it...to embrace economic realities than to battle them. The great success of our leadership will be to answer the question: "Which comes first in health care, price or quality???" Others have said that leaders do the right things and managers do things right. I would submit that in the 21st century quality leadership will be based on doing the right thing *and doing it right*. To survive and thrive in 2001 and beyond, nurse leaders must: Be there! Be vigilant! Be visible! Be helpful! Be smart! and Be honest!

The organizations in which we work, whether they are hospitals or community centers, will be vastly different from the ones we grew up in.

ORGANIZATIONS   Table 16

NEW		OLD
Dynamic Learning	→	Stable
Info.-Rich	→	Info. Scarce
Global	→	Local
Small & Large	→	Large
Customer Oriented	→	Functional
Skills-Oriented	→	Job Oriented
Team Oriented	→	Indiv. Oriented
Involvement Oriented	→	Controlled
Lateral Networked	→	Hierarchial

This means that the motivated leader in nursing will willingly recognize the nurse employee's talents. S/he will help the nurse to develop those exposed and under exposed talents. The nurse leader will not ignore weaknesses, but will not dwell on them either because they recognize that nurses are not children. They will use situational leadership to seek out and solve problems. There will be no sense or need to blame, only the need to be solution oriented. Finally the nurse leader of the 21st century will be honest, trustworthy, and straightforward. Because s/he knows h/his credibility will be based on sharing the big picture with empowered team members, being generous with information, praising frequently, and encouraging feedback.

The nurse leader's appraisal will be based on his or her credibility as involved in: the track record; enthusiasm; being informed; being relevant; and recognizing that nonverbal cues are more important than verbal cues. Passion is boundless enthusiasm; and the mandate for leadership will be to be boundlessly enthusiastic, flexible, and agile, especially in promoting open communication by being credible, by being concrete, and by being empathic.

LEADERS = OPEN COMMUNICATIONS BY:

1. BEING CREDIBLE
2. BEING CONCRETE
3. BEING EMPATHIC

"The winners of tomorrow will deal proactively with chaos. We'll look at the chaos per se as the source of market advantage, not as a problem to be got around" (Peters, 1987).

This is the real challenge for nurse leaders in the 21st century: to deal effectively with chaos in the new age of empowered nurses.

Chapter Eleven

BUYING INTO BUSINESS INTUITION

PART ONE

Intuition is knowledge gained without rational thought. Is there any nurse who has not at one time said, "You know I don't know how I know this, but...?" We know that women's intuition is really not what we are talking about. We're talking about a gut feeling called intuition which women and men who are nurses (and other kinds of people too) can have.

"Top down" leadership is not where nursing is heading today. We are moving into a time of true transformation in leadership structure. The old managerial styles (centralized management, hierarchial, distrust, rigidity, equity in pay, rational decision-making, formal communication, deep personalization, and striving for survival) are dead.

Today we are moving into a time of fewer nurses in hospital practice, most of whom will be in leadership roles. Self-managing teams will place all nurses in leadership roles. As a matter of fact, the sooner we stop using management as the context for describing what we do, the sooner we will all accommodate to what is transformational, and what must become a "bottom-up" approach for empowerment.

I believe that only then will we give up our dedication to "administrivia". In business for many years, managers and leaders have had administrative assistants. Some nurse managers have staffing coordinators who are not nurses. Some have even given up the prerogative of the manager to have the schedule done exclusively by that manager, letting somebody else do the schedule or even allowing nurses to do self-scheduling. Imagine that! Incredible!!

Table 17

MANAGEMENT BY INTUITION
1. "Non Desk" Thinking
2. Make a request of one's subconscious mind
3. Ask subconscious to work on a problem while sleeping
4. Experiment with "Inner Listening"
5. Self-talk (affirmations)
6. Self-Suggestion (refer all choices to the subconscious)

Duffy of the comics strips asks, "Do you have anything to show for the economic explosion of the 80s?" He says "Yeah, shrapnel wounds." As a matter of fact, nursing has much more than shrapnel wounds to show. It has been said that the 90's are penance for the 80's. This could be good news for nurses. We have bandaged our wounds in nursing for too long; and now in the mid- 90's, we're going to reconcile ourselves to a new type of leadership...the likes of which we have never experienced before. A featured part of that will be recognizing nurses at the practice level as very intelligent people, capable of extraordinary, intuitive action. Hallelujah!

Transformational leadership will result in semi-autonomous work units, decentralization, empowerment of nurses at the practice level, and trust and openness from the very beginning. Versatility and resilience on the part of every practicing nurse is critical. Payment for performance means that merit pay will be standard. An informal culture will be the heart of nursing. No longer will we tolerate a rigid culture that can't be breached without a ladder; but an informal culture characterized by respect, and caring by nurse executives, and by the nurses at the practice level. All of them striving for excellence up and down the ladder, to meet the client's needs in the most collaborative manner.

Ziggy, the great comic philosopher, asks "You are here, but where am I?" And that's my message on business intuition. Where are you? How much are you willing to give up in order to take on the new stressors of the late 1990s? Use intuition in transformation...or lose the advantage it provides.

Leadership has awkward beginnings. Very few nurses are prepared to be leaders/managers. All nurses, of course, are managers of client care and we do that very well. But usually nurses are selected for managerial positions because they were good nurses, not because they were good leaders. So once you get over the shock of somebody thinking you are good enough to be a leader/manager because you were a good nurse, and you realize that staff nurses suddenly distrust you, you can begin to focus on the skills you need to learn and achieve as a leader. Loneliness is part of management and leadership at the beginning. You were part of the rank and file, and suddenly it really is lonely at the top; and you can't figure out why nobody is talking to you. After all, just yesterday you were the nurse they consulted on every problem. So there's a generic ingrained loneliness in the role. There are also disappointments that come from the rather consistent failures that every leader/manager experiences. The loss factor in leadership is very high today. As a matter of fact, even the best are winning only 40 % of the time. So 40 to 60 % achievement rating is probably an A+ rating. For leaders collegial support is often missing, and the higher you go, the lonelier and the less support you have. Nevertheless, transformational leadership is a broader and more satisfying role than the one in the old system of "Management".

When you are a first line manager you have support from inside the organization. Once you reach the director and vice presidential level, you often have to go outside of your particular organization for that kind of support.

Intellectual foresight is the ability to plan beforehand. It is based on one's ability to be intuitive and action-oriented. Can you get foresight before you have hindsight? Maybe not. Experience really is the best teacher. We need depth perception to look upward and outward, not just downward. Seek the mentoring necessary for your professional growth and success. Every leader in hospitals today has to look upward and outward...beyond the scope of nursing practice. That leader also needs to develop peripheral skills because everybody in the institution, who is in management, is looking to see how much territory s/he can encroach on to have more power. It is interesting that the more people you supervise, the more power you are supposed to have. But this has not been true in nursing until now.

We need to re-vision constantly. This is called re-ordering priorities. The continuum of growth for nurse managers/leaders, for nurse leaders, moves from unconscious inefficiency to conscious inefficiency and ultimately to conscious efficiency...over time. That is also the progression from nurse manager to transformational, empowering, intuitive leader.

Establishing your particular leadership style will likely take you right through the first ten years of your career in leadership. Do not worry if you do not become consciously efficient by your fifth year: but recognize that your style will evolve over time. In the past it was thought that one was either born a manager, born a leader, or one never became one. That of course, is absolutely untrue. Today it is readily acknowledged that you can change your style; and you can develop into the kind of leader you wish to be, based on the people who have mentored you, and those whom you wish to emulate. Style is something that develops over a long period of time, and is based on experience; and definitely goes through stages of re-development.

We need also to develop habits of productivity. Productivity is very action oriented and can also be intuitive. The people with whom we work, expect certain objectives to be met. First these must be articulated, and then we are expected to meet them. Knowing the mission, the values, and the vision of the organization for which we work is the first order of business. Communicating those to the people who will actually implement the vision statement and the values, at the practice level is the nurse leader's most important priority. It is interesting that in nursing, it is the job we have valued least in managers and must come, in my opinion, to value most in our leaders.

Leadership requires thick skin. If you are inclined to sell yourself short, you can't eliminate psychosclerosis in yourself. You must be able to eliminate psychosclerosis in yourself, before you can eliminate it in anyone else. So focus on your self-imposed invisible entrapments: recognize that you're going to live with a lot of anxiety; you're going to live with a lot of worry. But learn to manage the guilt so we can function without remorse. Problems are the staple of the leader/manager's job. Solving other peoples' problems is exactly what a leader/manager is hired to do. Examples of those problems: baby sitting problems; battered women etc. Is the manager to be the therapist? The answer is that the manager may not be the therapist, but s/he must help the nurse seek some form of "therapy." Many nurses think the manager/leader's job is very didactic and paper-oriented, when in fact the biggest part of the job is communication: primarily active listening with humane responses. Fortune magazine in 1993 said that "Emotionally it's easier to change when you're hemorrhaging." This reminds us that even though the '90s are fraught with anxiety, fraught with change, in a truly revolutionary crisis, the truth is that the people with whom we work, and the hospitals we work in are hemorrhaging as they change. If you happen to be very safely placed right now you are not safe. The hemorrhage is coming, get ready for it, because no hospital in the United States will escape. All health care providers must change and adapt with agility and flexibility until the hemorrhage stops.

The prediction is that 1000 hospitals will close in this country before the year 2000. Converting the nurses' mentality from how that works against them, to how they can make that work for them is a great challenge. The re-deployment of nurses from hospitals to the community, with connectedness to the medical center, is the challenge of the 90's.   These changes require learning how to be honest with ourselves first, so that we can be honest with others. I specify self-honesty for nurse managers/leaders because if you can be honest with yourself, you can then generate honesty with others. The rule is "Tell the truth, always tell the truth...even when the news is bad." Nurses are very intelligent people; and we can handle the truth. Be more curious than cranky about everything in your world. You must look at everything with enormous curiosity. You need to break your routines, get out of your rut, and make sure you convert yourself to a people-oriented person, even if it means homework and paperwork every night. Look at yourself before you look at anybody else; and look at yourself honestly from the practice nurse's eyes. What does s/he see? Self-assess! What do they see when they look at you?

Intuitive leaders must develop empathy because when we feel we are lost in the quagmire, it is easy to forget how others feel. Empathy says you know how others feel. Be friendly, but do not be a buddy. Invest in knowledge skills for yourself. If you do not yet work in a paperless hospital, you will, if you are under the age of 40. You must be computer literate. You don't need to know how to program the computer, but you need to know what the computer will do for you. You need to recognize that knowledge skills are more important in the 21st century than any academic degree.

Give yourself thirty minutes a day and absolutely hold to it...thirty minutes, by yourself, to think things through, to assess yourself, to promote self-knowledge, to promote self-honesty. The person who knows how will always have a job, but the person who knows why, will always be h/her boss. Without time to reflect, we do not develop the requisite intuitive skills.

Make some predictions for yourself. Make planned developments as you identify weaknesses in your transformational skills. Remember to smile, because it's really important to demonstrate that your light is on for the people with whom you work...even in the worst of times.

Significantly important for women leaders in nursing, is the recognition that business is a great game. There's lots of competition and fun, few rules, and you keep score with money. That is a winner's perspective. It is also, at this point in nursing's development, a dominantly male perspective.

I remember when I first became an administrator in a formal setting. The person who hired me was someone I had worked with in a previous environment for thirteen years. He was the director of human resources and he was in charge of collective bargaining, among other things. I remember that Bill told me that what he loved best about his job was negotiating contracts in a unionized setting. He said he liked it because it was a game. I knew right then that there was one significant difference between men and women. We, who are women, do not usually see bargaining or negotiating as a game. We do not see business as a game, and we do not see our jobs as a game. I would submit that business is a game; and acknowledging that can cause you to smile more often. It's hard to smile if you are saying to yourself, " I'm not sure I'm ready for this." So self-evaluation and self-honesty are inherently important in what we do as leaders. Positive self-talk regarding the development of business intuition helps too.

> **A performance formula to keep in mind is:**
> **Vivid imagination x repetition.**

Vivid imagination is what Walt Disney once called "imagineering." Repetition means doing it over and over again. This gives us the winner's edge, but for those of us who are female, it gives us the women's edge. It is generally conceded that women are by nature, intuitive...not that women are mind readers, but that they are able to gain knowledge intuitively. We can convert that energy to a relentless, persistence in personal self-growth. Vivid imagination means that highly intuitive people can visualize and simulate their futures. If we begin to use this gift intelligently and purposefully in terms of self-affirmation and frequent practice, we will be successful leaders. That doesn't mean that we will win 100 % of the time. Remember a 40 % winning history, in today's marketplace, is a very big score.

Chapter Twelve

BUYING INTO BUSINESS INTUITION

PART TWO

There are those who would say about business and leadership that luck has a lot to do with it. I don't believe in luck. Luck is the intersection of preparation and opportunity. It has been said that chance favors the prepared mind. The more prepared you are, the more likely you are to take advantage of every opportunity, and win. Winners see risk as opportunity; and this is a more inherently masculine trait than it is a female trait. Most women simply did not grow up this way. So, we are obligated to mentor and guide new nurse leaders in this new way. By the 21st century all nurse leaders must recognize that risk is inherently opportunistic, and we cannot be afraid.

There may be such a thing as bad luck. But good luck we make for ourselves, and let me give you a very specific example. In the 1950s, Sir Alexander Fleming, the developer of penicillin, was visiting the National Institutes of Health in Washington, D.C. A young scientist was showing Sir Alexander his lab and said to him, " Sir Alexander, I'd like to show you my lab because I want you to know that every time I come into this beautiful, spotless laboratory, I say to myself, 'What would Fleming have developed if he had had a lab like this?' And Fleming looked at him and said, "We both know it wouldn't be penicillin". Fleming, you will recall, was looking for an anti-infective. His discovery was not serendipity. They were culturing soil samples to find anti-infectives. The mold which landed on his petri dish was the combination of preparation and opportunity.

You cannot be successful in business today and plan to be safe instead of sorry. How do you make the right moves? My prescription for being willing to move in new directions is positive self-expectancy. No matter what: Wake up happy. Absolutely force yourself to be positive in your outlook. Use positive talk to create your own positive mental attitude. In your work, if there is not a reservoir of joy, it's not the job for you. See problems as opportunities, concentrate on opportunities, and find the good in everything. There is good in everything today, because in a revolution and a crisis, good things happen. Relax and be friendly. Expect the best, because nurses do rise to the level of expectation. Find a role model for yourself, even if that role model has to be outside of the organization in which you work. That role model can be of either sex. Somebody who is empathic with your issues. Most importantly, associate with winners and optimists.

High performance and accountability increase as our self-esteem increases. If we can tolerate losses and negatives without loss of self-esteem, we are willing to be accountable for our performance.

Change is noisy. If you can manage the noise, you can help other nurses who work with you to manage the noise. It is when change is not noisy that nothing will change. Without noise, the change will fail or it is pseudo-change. As long as "they" are talking about it there is a chance of success. Even when "they" are irritated about it, if "they" are talking about it there is a chance of success. Change is noisy and leaders as change-agents are noise makers.

The principle in being a change agent is "WIIFM." "What's in it for me?" Be very realistic about this, and you will be willing to begin a change by sharing with the people who will have to implement the change. This is realistic, and an absolutely honest assessment as regards answering the question, "Why should I change?" Because once you enter a formal leadership position you are dependent on others for the implementation of the required changes.

"Dynamic inaction" in managers and leaders is a mortal sin. Dynamic inaction is doing nothing, but doing it with style (Boren, 1982). People who work with us, expect us to make decisions. We can forgive mistakes, but we cannot forgive doing nothing, and never being able to make a decision. These dynamic inaction verbs were made up by James Boren and include the following: fuzzify; profundify; pizzasify; demeanorize; nincompoopsify. All of these verbs represent dynamic inaction, or doing nothing, but doing it with style.

Table 18

DYNAMIC INACTION*	
Fuzzify	
	Fuddle Muddle
Pompistrut	
	Fudget
Oppsify	
	Idiotoxic
Nincompoopsify	
	Intervoid
Boobliate	
	Memostraddle
Demeanorize	
	Pizazzify
Drivelate	
	Yesbut
Profundity	
	Hunkerfy
Zilchify	
Doing Nothing With Style!	

Remember, intuition is knowledge gained without rational thought. However, intuition can be a learned skill. "Eureka," which means "I found it" in Greek, is based on intuition and there are four steps in the "Eureka Concept:" preparation, incubation, illumination, and verification. Using these four steps one can acquire intuition as a learned skill. Right-brainedness is intuitive. It is knowing that something is right without being able to explain it. The development of intuition as a learned skill, means using a lot of "non-desk" thinking. Not sitting at your desk thinking, but putting yourself in other modes of thinking. It means making requests of your subconscious mind in a very specific way so that somebody who is left-brained thinks it's a silly thing to do. But it works because you are asking questions of a part of your brain that doesn't usually get used much.

Ask the subconscious to work on a problem while you are sleeping. It's amazing. Sometimes you wake up with new ideas. Experience inner listening, in absolute quiet, and pay attention to yourself. Using self-talk (affirmations, etc) and using self-suggestion will increase your choices and your communication with your subconscious. It works something like this: I have these choices and I'm going to work on it, sleep on it, and wake up tomorrow to see what's there...in my subconscious.

Figure 12

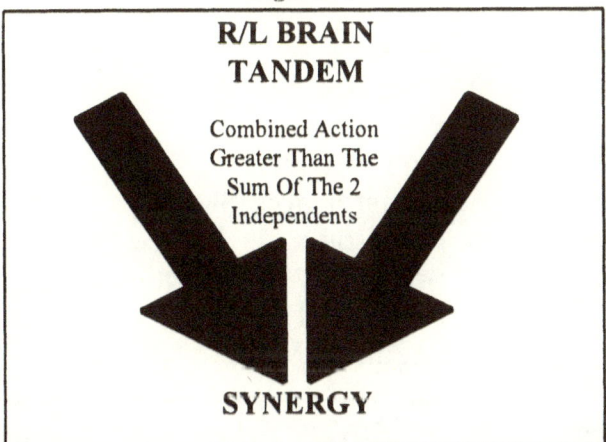

Steven Covey says, "The left brain is the monitor; the right brain is the mover." Covey has also written that to be principled leaders we need both sides of our brain (1989). To be effective leaders, to be principled leaders, we need to have both the monitor and the mover aspects of our brain working together. So the 1st step in the Eureka Concept is PREPARATION.

Table 19

```
EUREKA! (INTUITION)

1. Preparation
2. Incubation
3. Illumination
4. Verification
```

Preparation means setting goals and priorities and doing your homework. Use visualization and practice. Make absolutely sure that winning is a top priority. Make sure you have transferrable skills, people skills, and the didactic skills for monitoring. Use reflection in speaking to yourself too. By that I mean the old type of reflection that we learned a long time ago in psychiatric nursing to maintain open communication, this time with yourself. Preparation requires developing peripheral vision, asking for and welcoming feedback. It takes courage to ask for feedback, but preparation demands it.

Table 20

```
GO FOR IT: PREP

1. Set Goal & Priorities
2. Visualization
3. Practice
4. "Will to Win"
5. Transferrable Skills
6. Reflection
7. Sensitivity (personal radar)
8. Peripheral Vision
9. Feedback
```

The next step is INCUBATION. Incubation means allowing time for thoughts and feelings to settle. Go about your work, go about your business. Make sure that you begin with reflection, and develop alternatives: use a chart that allows for zigs and zags, pursue trial and error thinking. All of these are involved in the period of incubation. Use non-verbal imagery if you consider yourself a left-brained person. Develop the ability to think with the right side of your brain by forcing yourself to use non-verbal imagery. However, avoid analysis paralysis. People who are left-brained tend to go overboard and over analyze before they make decisions.

Table 21

INCUBATION

1. Reflection
2. Alternatives
3. Zigs & Zags
4. Pursue Trial & Error
5. Non Verbel Imagery
6. Avoid Analysis Paralysis
7. Avoid Parkinson's Law
8. Revoke Parato Principle
9. Use Imagination

Avoid Parkinson's Law which is, that work expands to fill the time available for it. Avoid making your work expand to fill all the time there is available for it. This is of the utmost importance for nurse leaders to learn. If you give someone two days to do the job, it'll take them two days to do a job. If it's your own business, you can get it done in ten minutes. Work expands to fill the time available for it.

Revoke the Parato Principle, which is that the trivial "stuff" takes up 80 % of the time, and important stuff only gets 20 % of the time. Make sure that you are giving 80 % of the time to "big stuff"; and 20 % of the time to trivia. Use your imagination to offset your tendency to rationalize.

After incubation there will come a period when you say, "Eureka! I have found it!" which, in this particular model, is called ILLUMINATION. Illumination arrives after incubation... from internal dialogue and listening...from trusting your hunches. Remember, a hunch is something trying to tell you something else. You just have a "feeling". Stop questioning yourself, stop questioning your qualifications. If you have the job, somebody thought you were good enough to have the job. Let your mind play and play yourself. In this health care crisis there will be many more failures than there are wins, but remember failure isn't fatal, and risking is being willing to make a mistake in an attempt to make progress. Listen to yourself and see the illumination.

Table 22

AH HA: Illumination

1. Listening To Yourself
2. Trusting Your Hunch
3. Stop Questioning Your Qualifications
4. Playing
5. Risking (failure is not fatal)
6. Fearing
7. Heeding Your Dreams
8. Turning Around Adversity
9. Timing

Give up fearing the unknown. Intuition is knowledge gained without rational thought...learn to trust it. Fear, uncertainty and doubt form our FUD Factor. I think the FUD Factor is common to all nurses who are female. Heed your dreams, heed your mentors, be willing to move in new directions. Turning things around means interpreting trends so that you see them differently. To get over my uncertainty, my fear, and my doubts I make a list of what could happen. If there are more good things than bad things on the list, I'm willing to risk it.

The last step in the Eureka Concept is VERIFICATION. You have to verify your illumination to make sure it wasn't just wishful thinking. Check it out with your support system. Don't be afraid to back down if your verification indicates that it was wishful thinking. Rehearse your presentation, rehearse your evaluation, and if you're in for a difficult time, rehearse every aspect of your communication. Stay tuned for new ideas because even if this illumination cannot be verified, something may grow out of it. Something you could not originally anticipate. Allow these to ripen. Give your ideas time to flower. Even if you are not successful this time, keep track of it. The proof is in the product: ultimately something will be achieved. Remember: the concept is not the only thing you are looking for. You are looking for implementation, and that's business by intuition.

Table 23

```
┌─────────────────────────────────┐
│        VERIFICATION             │
│                                 │
│  1. Avoid Wishful Thinking      │
│  2. Support Systems             │
│  3. Backing Down                │
│  4. Rehearsing                  │
│  5. Staying Tuned               │
│  6. Ripening                    │
│  7. The Proof = The product     │
│     or Concept                  │
│                                 │
│        MBI                      │
└─────────────────────────────────┘
```

Management By Intuition

Right-brained dominance can be developed, but it takes practice. If you know you are not highly intuitive, allow time for reflection, because left-brained people are very task-oriented, very analytical. Right-brainedness requires seeing your dreams, generating alternatives, allowing intuition time to grow. Doing jigsaw puzzles can help you get into your right brain. Be very future-oriented, because if you do develop your right brain, you can become more creative, more kinesthetic, or feeling in orientation and responsiveness to people. Left-brained dominance loves step by step procedures, loves concrete problem solving, loves monitoring, loves plotting, loves analysis. So our purpose is to get right and left brain intuition working in tandem.

Synergy is what we're looking for. Synergy, if we get the right and left brain working together, means that we will have a greater combined action of the two working together, than we'll ever have of the right brain working separately from the left brain. One and one is equal to three today. That's synergy. More productivity than from the simple sum of the two parts.

So: you manage from the left; but you lead from the right. Managers are said to do things right. Leaders are said to do the right things. So when I discovered the principle of the Eureka Concept, I knew I had one good reason for working at developing my right brain. You see I'm not over

73

fond of management, but I love the idea of leadership. I concluded, as a good left-brained person would, that I'd never be a great leader, if I didn't work on my right brain. I could always depend on my support system to giveme their right brain, but suddenly that wasn't good enough. It was only a substitute. Intangible skills for leaders and managers come from the right side of our brains: beliefs, ideals, decision-making, judgement, integrating skills, political savvy, and vision.

The left brain skills are the ones we have always worked with...the tangible skills: planning, coordinating, directing. We're trying to move into the right brain because we know we already have the left brain part solidly in place.

Why is this important? Why is intuition important? Because the fairy godmother is not coming!! As a leader, sometimes you feel like the pigeon, and sometimes you feel like the statue. Sometimes you feel like the statue because organizations have not learned to "F" themselves, which means to be fit, to be fast, to be focused and to be flexible. If you learn to "F" yourself, you will more often feel like the pigeon. Blessed are the flexible, they will not be bent out of shape!!...and they use both sides of their brain.

CHAPTER THIRTEEN

Working The System Of Shared Governance

In the late 20th century the social revolution of women's roles has increased opportunities for professional growth. These opportunities have brought to the professional nurse of today better education, more outspokenness, more self-assuredness, and less willingness to assume a dependent handmaiden role. This defines an interest in shared governance for the registered nurse. There are serious health care trends being established in this country that will last the rest of our careers. The idea of reducing health care expenditures is going to be here, irrespective of what reform the federal government ultimately decides on.

The focus for nurses, for the foreseeable future, will be cost, quality and service in nursing care. The mission, the vision, and the values of every health care agency which is to survive beyond the year 2000 will be...caring. To be concerned with customer satisfaction, to align the individual medical center with physicians in partnership, to be responsible for the use of resources are part of our mission. We must be willing to change and innovate until we find the right mix. Nurturing and empowering nursing staff will be key to gaining new business in institutions that provide health care. Total commitment to customer satisfaction in hospitals means an empowered nursing staff. To help with that mission we need to embrace the Japanese industry's "shared fate ethic," which represents empowerment, and, to me, is a form of shared governance: where everyone is involved with and affected by the fate of the organization. And everyone employed understands that ethic, too. In other words, we are all in this together...we share a fate.

If nurses do not embrace the shared fate ethic, I fear that we will continue to have more organizational aversion than we have organizational awareness. Organizational awareness, is trust and openness in a culture of pride. As opposed to organizational aversion, which occurs when people employed by an institution feel undervalued, misunderstood, and feel that the institution that employs them frankly doesn't care about them as individuals. When that exists, organizational aversion is the result of any change process. Attitudes about change process are always difficult to assess, and difficult to maintain optimism over the long term. Informed pessimism leads to failure. The role of the leader in change is to maintain optimism, hopeful realism, and, ultimately, success.

Shared governance is similar to TQM (total quality management) or TQL (total quality leadership) or CQI (continuous quality improvement).

Shared governance forms an allegiance and an alliance with each of these very comfortably. They are not mutually exclusive. In a shared governance environment, where nursing staff is empowered to professional practice, the shift to quality happens. Those shifts are:

From mistrust to trust;

From betrayal to working together;

From competition to cooperation;

From excellence as an ideal to excellence as a reality.

Florence Nightingale said:

"Such a tempest has been brewed in this little pint pot as you could have no idea of; but I, like the ass, have put on the whining skin, and when I once have done that, I can bray so loud that I shall be heard, I am afraid, in England. However, this is no place for lions, and as for asses, we have enough" (Ulrich, 1992). I couldn't agree more with Florence Nightingale. Let us move on. It has been said by many that crises can equal opportunity. In my experience, there are six phases to every project I have ever undertaken or been involved with during any crisis. Those six stages are: enthusiasm, followed by disillusionment, followed by panic, followed by a search for the guilty, followed by punishment of the innocent, and finally, followed by reward and honor for those who did *not* participate. These stages represent the antithesis of shared governance and professional practice. The decade of the 1990s will see the end of bureaucracy as we have known it in business and other forms of industry.

"The bureaucratic organization is becoming less and less effective,...it is hopelessly out of joint with contemporary realities, and...new shapes, patterns, and models are emerging which promise drastic changes in the conduct of the corporation and in managerial practices in general. So within the next 25-50 years, we should all be witness to, and participate in, the end of bureaucracy and the rise of new social systems better able to cope with 20th and 21st century demands" Warren Bennis.

"Any company that's going to make it in the 1990s and beyond has got to find a way to engage the mind of every single employee. If you're not thinking all the time about making every person valuable, you don't have a chance. What's the alternative? Wasted minds? Uninvolved people? A labor force that's angry or bored? That doesn't make sense!" John Welch, Jr.

It is clear then, that such radical changes in the nature of work are revolutionizing the entire modern society, and this must include nurses in health care delivery. All institutions are changing the relationships between employee and employer, between woman and man. After decades of narrow focus, employees, including nurses, are being asked to consider the whole, to innovate and care for customers, to work in self-governing teams, to figure out their own jobs; and to coordinate with others rather than just follow orders. The time of solving problems at the lowest level for customer satisfaction is upon us.

Thus, hierarchical ideas and behaviors are giving way to egalitarian beliefs and practices. In nursing this is epitomized in shared governance and professional practice. Responses must be directed by the point of impact, rather than from the point of power in nursing and all other industries. The basic role of each nurse in every health care organization, is changing. Shared governance is one way of re-engineering this essential transformation. As a leadership strategy, shared governance encourages, and even expects participation. It also promotes working conditions that encourage the individual nurses to work to their full potential. As a management approach, shared governance requires leadership over management; and mandates changes in every role along the traditional hierarchy.

Table 24

Traditional Hierarchy
- Follow directions
- Follow the chain of command
- Do the job...don't complain
- Don't make a mistake

Shared Governance
- Ask the question
- Make a suggestion
- The days of "free bitching" are over
- Talk to whomever gets the job done
- Don't be constrained by titles or positions
- Be responsible for the environment
- Be customer driven
- Be focused on quality
- Be focused on service
- See mistakes as learning opportunities
  (Nies and Kingdon, 1990)

The rationale behind shared governance and professional practice in nursing is simple. As the rate of change increases, managerial control becomes more difficult. Therefore, it is critical to involve the professional registered nurse in self-managing teams, and in problem solving at every level throughout the organization. New technologies, rapid sophisticated

77

communications, and endless discoveries make for a nightmare in a bureaucratic hierarchy. Leaders must recognize that control principles are ancient history in nursing. They must rely on the registered nurse to supply the information needed, to make sure that the right action is taken at the point of service for the health care agency's customer. Many nurses grew up in the traditional hierarchy. Many nurses became leaders/managers within a traditional hierarchy. The guides under which they developed were very clear:

Table 25

In The Traditional Hierarchy
• Run a tight ship
• Keep the boss informed
• Punish mistakes
• Set your own style
• Follow the chain of command
• The boss decides
• Keep the troops in line
• The boss is always right
• Don't rock the boat

However, change is here to stay. No organization in the American society will be immune, and this certainly applies to the health care system. The health care system will need to be better and more effective than ever as it moves into a time of health care reform and competition such as we have never known. Shared governance is the process of involving, including, and empowering the registered nurse at the practice level.

In Shared Governance: Table 26

• Talk to those who do the work
• Embrace errors
• Give up control
• Be inclusive in style
• Encourage questioning
• Invite challenges
• Show the way by example
• Find out for yourself
• Use consensus decision making
• Respect everyone in the system
(Nies and Kingdon, 1990)

For the best results to happen to professional practice in a shared governance system, significant role shifts are necessary. Giving up control and assuming responsibility are difficult adjustments for nurses to make. Perfect harmony will be a process rather than a destination. The journey, in and of itself, is worthwhile. All members of the organization must live the spirit of shared governance for full transformation to occur. The transformation of the registered nurse's professional practice to a shared governance system requires patience, nurturing, and guidance from all leaders in the system. The tone of the environment within the system must also change for specific actions to occur. The spirit and tone of shared governance will occur over time, when all members are nurtured to feel support, during and after the change process.

Table 27

What Happens When It Works? When shared governance works:

- Management moves from directing, controlling, to coaching and facilitating
- Centralized responsibility is replaced with shared decision making and shared responsibility
- Hierarchial structures give way to loose interactive structures where teams replace divisions and sections
- Respect, cooperation and collegiality replace competition and conflict on the nursing unit
- Communication becomes open and free-flowing instead of only up and down the system
- Purpose and power are shared, understood, and accepted by everyone in the system
- Rules, policies and procedures are kept to a minimum
- Guidelines and principles steer the nursing department
- Flexibility assures that rules may be bent when appropriate to meet objectives and goals
- Frustration and burnout are replaced by commitment in its members
- Members are committed to each other and to quality service for their customers
- Responsibilities are taken seriously and shared by every member of the nursing staff
(Nies and Kingdon, 1990; Pinchot, 1993; Renesch, 1992).

The crisis of health care reform, and the revolution it has caused in health care delivery, can equal an opportunity for the development of professional practice for nurses within a shared governance system. Be patient with the process of development, because the crisis of development for professional practice in nursing is an opportunity for us, such as we have not experienced before: the crisis of confusion can help us find new directions; the crisis of conflict can help us reach consensus: the crisis of stress can help us find support systems that we never knew we had; the crisis of alienation can help us find positive self-regard; and the crisis of spirit can help us find our own work essence. This means that registered nursing in a shared governance system can at last find its own work spirit, its own empowerment, and its own professional stature, separate from, but complimentary to medicine.

Chapter Fourteen

CONFLICT IS INEVITABLE...BUT MANAGEABLE

Conflict in a revolution is an inevitable part of our complex and competitive nursing society. Whether it be in our personal relationships or in our professional interactions, each of us sees conflict in terms of our own ideas, our own opinions, and our own needs. Among nurses, conflict is not seen as a happy event in our daily work. Nurses have not yet learned that resolving conflict takes hard work and enormous perserverence. How do we learn to handle this pervasive professional condition?

These are the words most frequently associated with conflict: fight, avoid, anger, lose, pain, control, impasse, hate, destruction, loss, fear, wrong, doing, mistake, bad   (Weeks, 1992).

Conflict resolution simply means getting people to work together productively. This means that nurses must learn to strengthen their abilities to deal with differences among the people with whom we work. It means using skill to resolve disputes and frustrations; and to strengthen relationships... recognizing that if we do not

LEARN TO TALK IT OUT...OR
WE WILL CONTINUE TO ACT IT OUT.

Conflict is therefore not, inevitably, destructive, although it can cause distress. Wishing will never make it go away. Therefore, we must learn to manage conflict as an essential life skill, which is vital in today's nursing profession.

The definition of a team is that a team is a collection of individuals guided by a common purpose, striving for the same results, to:
1. Solve problems
2. Togetherness
3. Reduce conflict
4. Increase productivity
5. Promote a culture of success and pride (Mallory 1991)

Resolving conflict usually means uniting your team, so that common goals can be achieved. Uniting a team requires three steps:
Step 1 Identify common psychological needs of team members
Step 2 Establish limits and ground rules for participation in team activities
Step 3 Build cohesion among team members (Pinchot and Pinchot, 1993)

Most teams have commonalities in terms of participants. For example, in a team of eight members there will be four usual kinds of team members:

• The dominant member- the one who needs challenges and recognition; is hard driving, demanding, and forceful
• The influencer as team member- the charmer, the persuasive one, the generous and social one
• The balancer team member- the one who is patient, the mediator who sees all sides of an issue
• The loyalist team member- who is honest, trustworthy, and dutiful (the loyalist is the most rigid team member who likes things to generally stay the same) (Mallory, 1991)

Team members, to be productive, must know the "hot buttons" to avoid; and the "triggers" to avoid to achieve common purpose and problem solving. This means being willing to make problem solving a team effort; to correct problems immediately; and to consistently monitor morale to maintain objectivity.

Conflict resolution in team management usually involves several basic tactics:

• Be honest and open
• Feel and show respect
• Be unconditionally constructive
• Be willing to use the art of confrontation

• Do not flaunt your authority
• Be passionate (have boundless enthusiasm)

By the same token each team member requires care and concern. It is usual to expect that team members need:

• Survival
• Security
• Belonging
• Prestige
• Self-fulfillment (Mallory 1991).

These needs can be fulfilled by the team itself, if the members of the team are interested in fulfilling each other's personal and professional goals.   Self-managing teams are foundational for the future of nursing. The re-structuring of nursing and hospitals, and the concomitant re-

structuring of nurses requires that nurses understand self-managing team functions better than ever before. Winning teams need:
- Coaching
- Recruiting
- Strategy
- Celebrating
- Anticipating
- Training
- Selecting
- Developing
- Practice
- Critiquing
- Motivating

Without the concern and ongoing training and re-training that self-managing teams require, conflict will be the continuous result.

Happiness is not the absence of conflict, but the ability to cope with it!! Women are taught to avoid conflict. Nurses are taught that conflict means: compromise; authority; confrontation; power; tension. Depending on how a nurse sees conflict, her response to conflict can be: defensive; fighting; angry; avoidance; harmonizing; apologizing; abdicating; crying etc., etc., etc. When searching for causes of conflict, nurses, and women in the American society, need to address the following possible causes of conflict:
- Self
- Needs or wants
- Values
- Perceptions
- Assumptions
- Knowledge deficits
- Expectations
- Race differences
- Gender differences
- Willingness to learn from conflict
- Willingness to learn to negotiate in conflict
(Weeks, 1992; Tjosvold, 1993)

Since nurses are at this moment in time primarily female, and since nurses who are female in the American society frequently suffer from negaholism (referred to in an earlier chapter of this book), it is common for defensiveness to be the primary response to conflict. Defensiveness is least likely to occur when: the other person appears to be equal to you; when information is available and free-flowing; when people work together to resolve conflict; and when trust is demonstrated throughout the department and unit of nursing. As nurses begin to develop a conflict management strategy it will be crucial to remember the following:

1. No power struggles
2. No avoidance allowed
3. Conflict does not set the agenda
4. Avoid "awfulizing"
5. Confront projection (Hendricks, 1991).

There are various stages of conflict resolution. There are three kinds of conflict:
1) Daily events which are least threatening and easiest to manage;
2) Challenges which require more training to resolve and specific skills for intervening;
3) True battles in which intervention is necessary
(Hendricks, 1991).

Resolving daily event conflicts requires good listening skills and help in seeing the big picture. These kinds of conflict are frequently reactions or responses to specific situations; and identifying the points of agreement and disagreement is usually sufficient to work out the problem. This is the fulfillment of the rule: we either talk it out or we act it out, once again.   The conflicts which are challenges require the creation of a safe and neutral place where facts can be reviewed and the middle ground negotiated. The most difficult kinds of conflicts to resolve are those called battles, where an outside mediator is frequently needed to intervene appropriately. This is an essential difference in the three kinds of conflict, because in battles, the shift is in wanting to win, to wanting to hurt other participants. Logic and reason will not be effective in this conflict resolution; and clear goals and a sense of direction are critical. It is essential to re-direct energy and encourage skill development in everyone as solutions are sought (Hendricks, 1991; Weeks, 1992 and Tjosvold, 1993).   Destructive conflict is characterized by the habit of avoiding conflict, with frequent outbursts of shouting and fighting which exacerbates our cycle of destructive conflict. Remember, there are benefits to conflict and these are frequently forgotten in the throes of defensiveness. Benefits that result from conflict are: problem awareness; productivity; organizational change; personal development; self acceptance; psychological maturity; challenge; and sometimes even fun (Tjosvold, 1993).

Nurses must learn the skills of conflict resolution as basic in solving the problems inherent in health care delivery today. The stressors which are impinging on nursing practice at every level, increase conflict, and therefore increase the need for problem solution. These are some guides for action that nurses can use as bench marks, in developing their skill in managing conflict:
• Commitment to learning to manage conflict as a basic skill
• Discussing the art of confrontation with conflict partners
• Setting ground rules and guidelines for cooperative conflict
• Establishing trust via the exchange of ideas and opinions
• Giving useful and descriptive feedback on how you
  feel and how you see conflict developing
• A sense of humor in your relationships
• Avoid making fun of people's weaknesses
• Avoid "put owns"
• Reduce personal control issues via therapeutic intervention, as needed
(Hendricks, Tjosvold, Weeks).

Figure 13

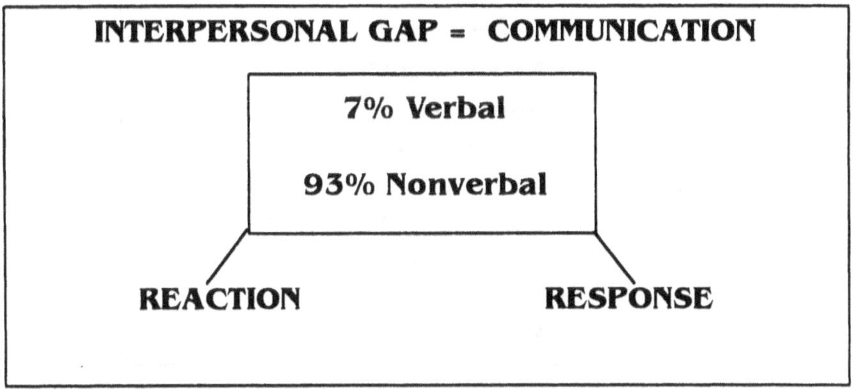

INTERPERSONAL GAP = COMMUNICATION

7% Verbal

93% Nonverbal

REACTION   **RESPONSE**

The essence of managing conflict in professional relation-ships **REQUIRES THAT YOU:**
• Create self-esteem; • Meet interpersonal needs; • Join the issue; invite discussion; and confront to heal!!

It is relatively easy to recognize one's own emotional response to conflict, since there are four immediate emotional responses to any conflict situation: blaming; secrecy; repressed feelings; and anger. The point in managing conflict effectively is to recognize one's own emotional response, and work toward effective resolution of the conflict through confrontation to heal and/or talking it out. It is important to understand that there have been persistent myths regarding conflict among nurses:1) conflict usually means poor management; 2) conflict usually means organizational aversion and organizational negativity; 3) conflict can be self-contained, and will take care of itself; 4) conflict always must be resolved (Hendricks,1991).

Myths are usually handed down by nurses from generation to generation, and do not represent fact or truth. Please review the list of persistent myths again, and remember: these are not necessarily truth and more likely are fiction.

Changes occur in individual nurses when conflict is managed successfully. There are specific growth characteristics which are identifiable in nurses who become posaholics instead of maintaining a negaholic behavior pattern.

Changes will occur in nurses when conflict is managed successfully

Table 28
Growth Characteristics for <u>Posaholics</u>

• **Self esteem ↑**
• **Accountability**
• **Optimism**
• **Imagination**
• **Creative**
• **Communication**
• **Committed**
• **Alert**
• **Aware**

When conflict is understood as inherent in the community in which we live or work, then it is possible to manage conflict in a mutually beneficial manner. These are the essential steps to managing conflict:

1) Create an atmosphere conducive to negotiation

2) Clarify individual perceptions

3) Develop a shared point of view

4) Focus on individual as well as shared needs

5) Believe in empowerment: share positive power

6) Make mutually beneficial agreements

Please note that none of the steps involves liking or loving each other in conflict resolution. Managing conflict does mean liking or loving *yourself* enough to confront another person with whom you have a conflict in a healing manner, so that the conflict is resolved. (Please see figure three for the satisfied participant in conflict resolution. Also note the two reminders which follow this paragraph).

REMINDER #1	REMINDER #2
Either we are together OR We are pulling apart	**COMMON COURTESY IS NOT COMMON!**

Conflict resolution/management begins when nurses recognize that "power garbage" has no place in the profession of nursing. Power garbage can be defined as the game nurses play with each other called, "Who is in charge?" When the power relationships which exist in nursing today become truly collegial, and shared empowerment is the norm, then the disease of powerlessness will leave the profession; and we will exist in a system that not only needs, but also advocates, self-managed teams in nursing. Effective team work means effective conflict management for all professional participants in nursing.

COMING TOGETHER IS A BEGINNING...STAYING TOGETHER IS PROGRESS...WORKING TOGETHER...IS SUCCESS!!!

There has never been a time in the American society of greater distress and greater change. Stress and change create conflict. Managing conflict successfully requires a positive mental attitude. Some significant reminders for maintaining a positive mental attitude:

WHAT IS LIFE?

Life is a gift...accept it. Life is an adventure...dare it. Life is a mystery...unfold it. Life is a game...play it. (Author Unknown)

AFTERWARD

We are rapidly developing new traditions in nursing. Impelled by societal changes and reforms in health care delivery, nurses are finding a new voice, and new roles. Our practice is knowledge based, confident, and full of the potential to be a full partner in a delivery system that emphasizes community and prevention.

THE PARABLE OF THE STARFISH

As an old man walked the beach at dawn, he noticed a young woman picking up starfish and flinging them into the sea. Finally, catching up with her, he asked her why she was doing this. The answer was that the stranded starfish would die if left in the morning sun. "But the beach goes on for miles and there are millions of starfish," countered the old man. "How can your effort make any difference?"   The young woman looked at the starfish in her hand and then threw it to the safety of the waves. "It makes a difference to this one," she said.

- Anonymous

Our value to society, as nurses, is based on our desire to make a difference and that depends on what we do with what we have in our professional practice.

REFERENCES

American Nurse (Washington,D.C.: The American Nurses Association, 1991, 1992, 1993, 1994).

Barrentine, P. (ed.), When The Canary Stops Singing (San Francisco: Barrett-Koehler, 1993).

Bean, W., Strategic Planning (Amherst, MA: HRD Press, 1993).

Bethel, S.M., Making A Difference (New York: Putnam, 1990).

Bohm, D., Wholeness and The Implicate Order (London: Ark Publications, 1980).

Boren, J., Fuzzify (McLean, Virginia: EPM Publications, 1982).

Bramson, R., Coping With Difficult People (New York: Anchur, 1981).

Carter-Scott, C., The Corporate Negaholic (New York: Villard, 1991).

Coile, R., The New Hospital (Maryland: Aspen, 1986).

Covey, S., The Seven Habits of Effective People (New York: Simon and Schuster, 1989).

Drucker, P., The Post Capitalist Society (New York: Harper, 1993).

Drucker, P., Managing For The Future (New York: Truman-Talley, 1992).

Drucker, P., " The Coming of The New Organization," Harvard Business Review, 1988, 66(5), 45-53.

Galbraith, J. et al., Organizing For The Future (San Francisco: Jossey-Bass, 1993).

Gasparis,L. and Swirsky, J., Nurse Abuse (New York: Power Publications, 1990).

Goodstein,L. et al., Applied Strategic Planning (San Diego: Pfeiffer, 1992).

Hammer, M. and Champy, J., Reengineering The Corporation (New York: Harper, 1993).

Hendricks, W., How To Manage Conflict (Shawnee, Kansas :National Press, 1991).

Kanter, R., The Change Masters (New York: Simon and Shuster, 1983).

Kanter, R., "The New Managerial Word," Harvard Business Review, 1989, 67:6 85-92.

Kubler-Ross, E., On Death and Dying (New York: Macmillan, 1969).

Larsen, E. and Goodstein, J., Who's Driving The Bus (San Diego: Pfeiffer, 1993).

Lathrop, J.P., Restructuring Health Care (San Francisco: Jossey-Bass, 1993).

Mallory, Charles, Team Building (Shawnee Mission, Kansas: National Press Publications, 1991).

Maynard, H. and Mehrtens, S., The 4th Wave (San Francisco: Barrett-Koehler, 1993).

Modern Health Care (Chicago: Crain Pubications, 1992, 1993, 1994).

Naisbitt, J. and Aburdeen, P., Megatrends 2000 (New York: Avon, 1990).

Nies, M. and Kingdon, R., Leadership in Transition (Illinois: Nova Ltd, 1990).

Nolan, T. et al., Shaping The Organization's Future (San Diego: Pfeiffer, 1993).

Perlman, D. and Takacs, G., "The Ten Stages of Change," Nursing Management 21, No.4: 1990.

Peters, T., Thriving on Chaos (New York: Knopf, 1987).

Peters, T., Seminar (New York: Vintage, 1994).

Pinchot, G and Pinchot, E., The End Of Bureaucracy (San Francisco: Barrett-Koehler, 1993).

Renesch, J.(ed.), New Traditions In Business (San Francisco: Barrett-Koehler, 1992).

St Exupery, A., The Little Prince (New York: Harcourt, Brace and Jovanovich, 1973).

Tagliere, D., How To Meet, Think, and Work To Consensus (San Diego: Pfeiffer, 1992).

Tjosvold, D., Learning To Manage Conflict (New York: Lexington Books, 1993).

Toffler, A., Power Shift (New York: Bantam Books, 1990).

Ulrich, B., Leadership and Management According To Florence Nightingale (Norwalk, Connecticut: Appleton & Lange, 1992).

Van Oech, R., Creative Whack Pack (Stamford, Connecticut: U.S. Games Systems, 1988).

Vogt, S. and Murrell, K., Empowerment in Organizations (San Diego: Pfeiffer, 1990).

Weeks, D., Conflict Resolution (New York: G.P. Putnam, 1992).

Wooten, P., Presentation at a meeting of The National Nurses in Business Association, San Francisco, 1992.